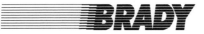

Prehospital Care of the Elder Patient

Robert A. Partridge, MD, MPH, DTM, FACEP
Rhode Island Hospital

Bruce M. Becker, MD, MPH, FACEP
Rhode Island Hospital

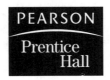

PEARSON
Prentice
Hall

Upper Saddle River, New Jersey 07458

Library of Congress Cataloging-in-Publication Data

Partridge, Robert A.

  Prehospital care of the elder patient / Robert A. Partridge, Bruce M. Becker. —
1st ed.

      p. cm.

Includes bibliographical references and index.

  ISBN 0-8359-5192-8

  1. Medical emergencies. 2. Geriatrics. 3. Aged—Medical care. I. Becker,
Bruce M. II. Title.

RC925.5.B43 2003

618.97—dc21

Publisher: Julie Levin Alexander
Publisher's Assistant: Regina Bruno
Senior Acquisitions Editor: Tiffany Salter
Editorial Assistant: Joanna Rodzen-Hickey
Senior Marketing Manager: Katrin Beacom
Channel Marketing Manager: Rachele Strober
Director of Production and Manufacturing: Bruce Johnson
Managing Production Editor: Patrick Walsh
Manufacturing Buyer: Pat Brown
Production Liaison: Julie Li
Production Editor: Karen Ettinger, The GTS Companies/York, PA Campus
Creative Director: Cheryl Asherman
Cover Design Coordinator: Christopher Weigand
Cover Designer: Kevin Kall
Cover Image: Photodisc
Compositor: The GTS Companies/York, PA Campus
Printer/Binder: R.R. Donnelley & Sons
Cover Printer: Coral Graphics

Credits and acknowledgments borrowed from other sources and reproduced, with permission, in
this textbook appear on appropriate page within text applicable.

Pearson Education LTD.
Pearson Education Singapore, Pte. Ltd
Pearson Education, Canada, Ltd
Pearson Education—Japan

Pearson Education Australia PTY, Limited
Pearson Education North Asia Ltd
Pearson Educación de Mexico, S.A. de C.V.
Pearson Education Malaysia, Pte. Ltd

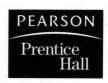

10 9 8 7 6 5 4 3 2 1
ISBN 0-8359-5192-8

This book is dedicated to my wife, Karen, and our children, Rachel, Sarah, and Alexander, for their love, patience, encouragement, and understanding.

RAP

I dedicate this book to my grandparents, Elsie (1912–2001) and Harold Weiss (96 years old and still energized!), who lived to celebrate their 75th wedding anniversary and taught me that dignity, wisdom, and love only grow with each passing year!

BMB

Contents

Preface

This book was written to address a glaring deficit in the prehospital literature. In reviewing the many books available for teaching emergency medical technicians and paramedics for our own courses, we found none that focused on prehospital care of the elder patient. Elder patients represent a considerable proportion of all patients treated and transported by prehospital emergency medicine personnel. Yet not only are no texts devoted to this important subject, but a review of current standard prehospital textbooks also reveals almost no information at all that specifically addresses older patients.

We undertook this project to educate prehospital emergency medicine personnel about the assessment, stabilization, and management of this important and expanding patient group. It focuses specifically on issues affecting older patients and on how prehospital management of these patients differs from that of other cohorts. This book is intended for all emergency medical technicians at the basic level, with additional advanced material in each chapter geared toward the paramedic level. Each chapter also includes a question set for self-assessment and review. Prehospital providers at all levels can benefit from the information in this text and easily apply this knowledge to their specific situations.

Section One of this book is intended to provide a general introduction to the management of the prehospital patient. It focuses on the differences between elder patients and other adult patients whom the emergency medical technicians or paramedics encounter in the course of their practice. Key topics include the changing anatomy, physiology, and pathophysiology of the elder patient, and how these changes affect the work of the prehospital provider.

Section One also focuses on the assessment of the elder patient. It is divided into two subsections: 1) assessment of the elder patient with medical illness, and 2) assessment of the elder patient who has suffered trauma. As in other patients, assessment is grounded in the ABCs (airway, breathing, circulation), but it must be adapted to the particular presentation of the elder patient, who very often provides a confusing picture to prehospital emergency personnel, as well as to the medical staff at the emergency department. Problems that are easily diagnosable in other patients, such as shock, myocardial infarction, and acute abdominal emergency, are often masked and present in an occult fashion in the elder patient. It is essential for the prehospital provider to be cognizant of these differences in presentation and take them into account in deciding on initial stabilization and approach to these patients. The elder trauma patient also can be very difficult to assess. Baseline changes in cognition, multiple cardiac and other medications, and long-standing chronic disease may interfere with the normally adequate trauma evaluation.

The management of medical emergencies is the focus of Section Two, which reviews medical considerations specific to elder patients, including cardiovascular, pulmonary, gastrointestinal, genitourinary, neurological, endocrine, toxicological, environmental, and behavioral pathology and pathophysiology. This hands-on review is very symptoms and systems based, stressing basic strategies for assessment, stabilization, and transport. The paramedic section goes into greater depth in each of the medical subsections in order to broaden and deepen the paramedics' understanding of these problems in the elder patient.

Section Three examines trauma in the elder patient, with a focus on assessment of the cardiovascular system, shock, bony, and neurological injuries. Perception of pain, ability to communicate, and lowered baseline level of functioning can interfere with appropriate assessment and intervention in elder trauma patients. It is quite common to underestimate the degree of injury. For an elder patient, even a minor fall can result in a fracture or contusion of the liver or spleen, with extensive intraperitoneal hemorrhage. This section offers specific guidance for avoiding pitfalls in evaluating these patients.

In Section Four the pharmacological management of the elder patient is reviewed. The first part of this section delineates differences in the absorption and metabolism of medication in the normally functioning elder person, and then addresses specific organ system dysfunction as it affects medications. The second part of the section reviews specific medications and considerations for their use in elder patients.

Section Five focuses on the medicolegal aspects of care of the elder patients. Very often, prehospital providers find themselves on difficult legal and ethical ground when trying to decide whether to initiate full or critical care in the acutely ill or dying elderly patient. Often, relatives disagree about the wishes of the patient, the presence or absence of living wills or other documents, and the contents of those documents. This section also addresses neglect and abuse, a growing problem in the United States. The prehospital provider has both a medical and a legal obligation to report any suspicions of neglect and abuse, but the signs are often very subtle. Often, clues picked up by the prehospital emergency medicine practitioner from the patient's home environment provide some of the only information the physician or nursing staff can use to begin an investigation of neglect or abuse.

It is our sincere hope that this text on prehospital care of elder patients will be an important addition to the growing body of knowledge for prehospital care providers. The ultimate goal of this project is to enhance the ability of prehospital providers to care for elder persons.

ACKNOWLEDGMENTS

We would like to thank the reviewers who provided invaluable comments and suggestions. They are Brenda Beasley, RN, BS, NREMT-P, Calhoun College; Danny Bercher, MEd, NREMT-P, University of Arkansas for Medical Sciences; Christopher Black, Eastern Arizona College; Debra Cason, University of Texas Southwestern Medical Center; JoAnn Cobble, University of Arkansas for Medical Sciences; Richard G. Fuller, Beattie Technical School-Public Safety; Jonathan Scott Hartlley; David J. Kuchta, RN, NREMT-P, BSAS, Advanced Life Support Coodinator; John S. Molnar, Cleveland Clinic Health System; Dawn W. Orgeron, RN, NREMT-P, EMS Administration, NOHD EMS; Elisa M. Reeves, NREMT-P, First Response Medical Training, LLC; Robert K. Waddell, II, EMSC National Resource Center; and Judith L. Warren, PhD, Texas A&M University.

Robert A. Partridge, MD, MPH, DTM, FACEP
Department of Emergency Medicine
Rhode Island Hospital
Assistant Professor of Medicine (Emergency Medicine)
Brown University School of Medicine
Providence, RI

Bruce M. Becker, MD, MPH, FACEP
Department of Emergency Medicine
Rhode Island Hospital
Associate Professor of Medicine and Community Health
Brown University School of Medicine
Providence, RI

Contributing Authors

Robert Partridge MD, MPH, DTM, FACEP, FAAEM
Assistant Professor of Medicine
Brown University School of Medicine
Department of Emergency Medicine
Rhode Island Hospital
Providence, RI
(EDITOR)
(Environmental Emergencies, Elder Abuse and Advance Directives)

Bruce Becker, MD, MPH, FACEP
Associate Professor of Community Health
Brown University School of Medicine
Department of Emergency Medicine
Rhode Island Hospital
Providence, RI
(EDITOR)
(Introduction and Assessment of the Elder Patient)

Robert H. Woolard, MD, FACEP
Chairman, Department of Emergency Medicine
Associate Professor of Medicine
Brown University School of Medicine
Rhode Island Hospital
Providence, RI
(Section Editor, Medical Chapters)

Mara Stankovich Aloi, MD
Clinical Instructor
Department of Emergency Medicine
MCP Hahnemann University School of Medicine
Allegheny General Hospital
Pittsburgh, PA
(Abdominal Emergencies)

Kevin A. Osgood, MD, FAAEM, FACEP
Emergency Physician
Seneca, SC
(Cardiac Emergencies)

Rebecca Bollinger-Parker, MD
Assistant Professor of Emergency Medicine
Texas Tech University Health Sciences Center at El Paso
Assistant Medical Director
Thomason Hospital Emergency Department
El Paso, TX
(Psychiatric and Behavioral Emergencies)

Brian J. Wilson, NREMT-P
Education Director
Texas Tech University Health Sciences Center at El Paso
Division of Emergency Medical Services
El Paso, TX
(Psychiatric and Behavioral Emergencies)

John E. Morley, MB, BCh
Division of Geriatric Medicine
Saint Louis University Health Sciences Center
Geriatric Research, Education and Clinical Center
St. Louis VA Medical Center
St. Louis, MO
(Endocrine Emergencies)

Masood Khan, MD
Costal Family Health Center
Bay St. Louis, Mississippi
(Endocrine Emergencies)

Jonathan Valente, MD
Fellow in Pediatric Emergency Medicine
Jacobi Medical Center
Albert Einstein College of Medicine
Bronx, New York
(Toxicologic Emergencies)

David C. Lee, MD, FAAEM
Director of Research
Department of Emergency Medicine
North Shore University Hospital
Manhasset, NY
(Toxicologic Emergencies)

Selim Suner, MD, MS, FACEP
Assistant Professor of Surgery
Brown University School of Medicine
Department of Emergency Medicine
Rhode Island Hospital
Providence, RI
(Musculoskeletal Trauma, Abdominal Trauma)

Alexander Lee, MD
Attending Physician
Department of Emergency Medicine
Doctors Community Hospital
Lanham, MD
(Chest Trauma)

Liudvikas Jagminas, MD, FACEP
Assistant Professor of Surgery
Brown University School of Medicine
Department of Emergency Medicine
Rhode Island Hospital
Providence, RI
(Head and Neck Trauma)

Lawrence Proano, MD, DTM
Clinical Associate Professor of Surgery
Brown University School of Medicine
Department of Emergency Medicine
Rhode Island Hospital
Providence, RI
(Pharmacology)

John F. Jardine, MD
Department of Emergency Medicine
Falmouth Hospital
Falmouth, MA
(Neurologic Emergencies)

Kyle B. McClaine, MD
Attending Physician
Department of Emergency Medicine

The William W. Backus Hospital
Norwich, CT
(Genitourinary Emergencies)

Mark Williams, MD
Attending Physician
Department of Emergency Medicine
Kaiser Foundation Hospital
Hayward, CA
(Pulmonary Emergencies)

SECTION I

Introduction

1

The Prehospital Provider
and the Elder Patient

Bruce Becker, MD, MPH, FACEP

OBJECTIVES

By the end of this chapter, the prehospital health care provider should be able to:

1 Identify the challenges elder patients present to the prehospital provider.

2 Determine the extent to which the elderly use the Emergency Medical Services (EMS) system compared with other age groups.

3 Introduce and discuss the special medical, traumatic, and psychosocial needs the elder require of the prehospital provider.

CASE

You are called to transport a patient. She cannot or will not communicate except in loud, obnoxious, repetitive vocalizations, grunts, and screams. She has no teeth and spits up partially digested food on anyone who gets close to her. She cannot ambulate and must be carried, but whenever a stranger tries to move her, she cries and tries to wriggle out of their grasp. She will not listen to reason and becomes inconsolable, kicking and yelling. You are told that she has a sleep disorder and often awakens the entire household several times a night. Her caregivers look exhausted. She is incontinent of urine and stool, and cannot attend to her most basic personal needs.

Can you picture this patient? Have you seen any patient like this in the last year? How would you feel about taking care of her? Would you be empathic, concerned, excited, filled with a sense of hope and caring? What if I told you she was eight months old? We health care workers have preconceived notions, prejudices, and stereotypes. There are types of patients who we like to take care of and others that we shy away from, pay less attention to, or write off. We make preliminary judgments about their quality of life, and even their ability to perceive and respond to our input, our care, and our touch. Our summary judgments reflect on us and are a result of our culture, our upbringing, and the societal values that surround us.

Americans in the new millennium appear to place more value on youth, youthful appearance, beauty, and physical vigor, and less importance on the social, physical, and medical decline that seems inevitably to be associated with growing old. This viewpoint is held by many health care professions as well. Samuel Shem's novel *The House of God* coined the pejorative term *GOMER* (Get Out of My Emergency Room), referring to an elderly, usually demented, patient with many chronic and unresolvable medical problems, on multiple medications, who has had dozens of hospital admissions generating a medical record spanning several volumes. We have all been guilty at one time or another of using the word *GOMER* or a similarly disparaging equivalent to refer to an elder patient who we preferred not to care for. If you work for a reasonably busy EMS system, you probably care for elder patients almost every day. Next time you care for such a patient, stop and reflect on the following:

Every GOMER could be someone's grandmother or grandfather. That patient raised children and grandchildren, and those people love and respect the patient, just like you love and respect your parents and grandparents.

You, too, if you are lucky, and choose a healthy lifestyle, will be a GOMER someday. Will some disrespectful, short-sighted health care worker be as easily willing to disregard your whole life of accumulated experiences and wisdom just because you are old and not physically or mentally robust?

When many people think about the elderly, the image of a bed-bound nursing home patient comes to mind. However, the truth is that most elderly people are active and independent, and many enjoy life more than when they were younger. Even people in their 80s or older are out fishing, camping, traveling, exercising, and participating in numerous recreational and work activities. Prehospital health care providers are often called to provide emergency care for these elders as well. A good working knowledge of the health care problems of the elderly ensures the best care of these patients.

Elder persons are the fastest growing segment of the population, and the fastest growing segment of the elder population are those 85 and older. More than 15 percent of Emergency Department visits are made by elders. They are four times more likely than non-elders to use ambulance and rescue services for transport to the emergency department and five times more likely to be admitted to the hospital once they have arrived there. Almost 20 percent of elders will use prehospital services in the next year. They are your most frequent and best customers. They are also your most challenging patients.

Prehospital emergency care is physically and psychologically uncomfortable and stressful for elders. Privacy and modesty are important to elders, yet both are often disregarded by the health care system, beginning in the prehospital setting. In addition, elders have great fear about entering the emergency department or hospital. They are often trying desperately to maintain independence and control over their lives. Illness and injury can cause loss of independence and may initiate a series of events that lead to the nursing home, the intensive care unit, or death.

Elders often have many chronic medical problems, may take many different medications, may have limited functional reserve (i.e., their organs cannot compensate for the additional stress brought on by acute disease), may have difficulties with thinking and expressing their thoughts and needs, and may present with different and more subtle signs and symptoms than younger patients (even though they may have the same diseases). They can be difficult to evaluate, especially in the prehospital setting. Their medical problems are complex, and if acutely ill or injured, they can quickly decompensate, requiring advanced life support (ALS).

The appropriate and effective prehospital evaluation and treatment of elders demands a thorough, intelligent, caring approach by health care professionals who understand the complexities of their patients, the pitfalls that lurk behind even benign complaints, and the devastating consequences to the elder patient of improper care. This textbook was written to address the unique medical, traumatic, and psychosocial problems that the prehospital health care worker encounters when caring for elder patients. More commonly than with younger patients, the thoroughness and effectiveness of the prehospital intervention can determine the entire course and outcome of the emergency department visit and hospitalization for that patient.

The elder patient you are called to see must be treated with the same concern and thoroughness as the eight month old. Both demand your best skills. They are the bookends of our lives' stories. No story is complete without a beginning and an end. We all were once children, and most will be elders. Treat your elder patients with the respect you show for your grandparents, with the respect that you hope will one day be shown to you.

REVIEW QUESTIONS

1. The fastest growing segment of the U.S. population is
   a. newborn to age 5
   b. ages 6–18
   c. ages 19–64
   d. age 65 and older

2. Elder patients are _____ more likely than the younger population to activate the EMS system.
   a. two times
   b. four times
   c. six times
   d. eight times

3. What percentage of elders use the EMS system in a given year?
   a. 5 percent
   b. 10 percent
   c. 20 percent
   d. 50 percent

4. Elders who activate the EMS system are likely to fear all of the following *except*
   a. disturbing their neighbors
   b. lack of privacy
   c. loss of independence
   d. severe illness or death

2

Assessment of Ill or Injured Elder Patients

Bruce Becker, MD, MPH, FACEP

OBJECTIVES

By the end of this chapter, the prehospital health care provider should be able to:

1 Discuss the unique importance of scene assessment in the prehospital care of the elder patient.
2 Explain the A, B, C, D, and E of initial assessment, with particular attention to the special problems presented by the elder medical and trauma patient.
3 Discuss the four vital signs and special considerations for elders.
4 Discuss the importance of the history in the elder patient.
5 Review the focused assessment in detail for the elder medical or trauma patient.
6 Discuss special problems in stabilizing and transporting elder patients.

SCENE ASSESSMENT

Scene assessment in the prehospital management of the elder patient presents some unique challenges to the provider, and the information obtained on site can be invaluable to hospital-based caregivers who take over the care of the patient. The prehospital health care provider arriving on scene should first perform a brief survey of the scene itself to determine the mechanism of injury in the trauma patient, or the severity and type of illness in the medical patient. As is accepted practice, the prehospital health care provider should identify potential scene hazards to rescuers, adopt universal precautions, secure the scene, and locate the patient.

Elder patients may not be able to give an accurate history. If they have cognitive difficulties, they may not be able to give any sort of coherent history at all. It is imperative that the caregiver make every effort to obtain the history from other persons present at the scene. These may be family members, home health care aides, neighbors, or bystanders. These people may be the only ones with any knowledge of what has been going on with the patient just prior to the incident for which the emergency medical services (EMS) system was activated. Some of these people may be able to provide very important information that cannot be obtained from any other source. It may be that the primary care physician has not seen the patient for weeks or months, and has never visited the patient's home. The appearance, demeanor, and examination of the patient in a physician's office can be very different and not representative of the environment in which the patient lives.

If the patient is critically ill or injured, it may not be possible for the prehospital health care provider to complete the scene assessment prior to carrying out an initial assessment of the patient. Whenever possible, one prehospital health care provider should continue the scene assessment while the other initiates the primary assessment of the patient. The prehospital health care provider should get a sense of the patient's home environment. This is particularly important in the case of home trauma. Is the lighting adequate? Are there slippery rugs on the floor, or does the floor have a slick wooden surface? Are there fire hazards in the home? Does the patient or other home occupants smoke? What is the temperature of the home? This is especially important, because elder patients are much more susceptible to hypo- and hyperthermia. What sort of clothing was the patient wearing, and was it appropriate for the temperature of the environment?

Family members and other caregivers in the home that the prehospital health care provider may encounter may not be traveling to the hospital and may not be present to support or augment the patient's history. If possible, try to obtain information about the patient's medical problems, medications, medication compliance, diet, activities, mental status, and physical status in the few days leading up to the incident. Try to obtain the patient's medications and take them with you when you transport the patient to the hospital. Elder patients are often on multiple medications and frequently cannot remember all the medications they take. Bringing their medication list or a bag containing all their medications may be the only way that hospital personnel caring for the patient will know what medications have been prescribed for them. Remember that medications are expensive—reassure the patient that both you and the receiving hospital will keep their medications safe, like all patient belongings. If there are any medical records or paperwork accompanying the medications, include them with the medications that you are transporting. Make every effort to bring eyeglasses, hearing aids, and false teeth. These items can aid communication with the elderly patient; moreover, their absence will add to the patient's sense of confusion, fear, and disruption.

Note the condition of the home. Is it well kept and clean, or dirty and clearly not taken care of? This may reflect on the mental status or chronic physical condition of the patient, or the presence and attentiveness of the caregivers. Is there food in the refrigerator or cabinets? Elders sometimes have great difficulty in getting out to obtain food and may be severely malnourished because of their inability to obtain appropriate food to eat. Is there alcohol in the house, opened bottles of wine or liquor with glasses in the kitchen or in other rooms of the home? Alcoholism is not uncommon in elders and can be a major complicating factor of the elder's illness or injury. Alcoholism is not well recognized in elders by physicians or other health care professionals. Information that the prehospital health care provider brings with them to the hospital may be very important in assisting the physician or nurse to identify this treatable, but potentially fatal problem.

INITIAL ASSESSMENT

The initial assessment consists of the A, B, C, D, and Es, which stand for Airway, Breathing, Circulation, Disability, and Expose. As you have been taught many times before, the purpose of the initial assessment is to uncover and treat life-threatening conditions. As you perform the initial assessment, treat all life-threatening problems that you find. For example, if the patient does not have an airway, provide one prior to checking the breathing.

If your initial assessment reveals that the patient is conscious and alert, take a moment to remember some unique things about the elder patient. These patients may have underlying cognitive deficits. Even if their mental status is intact, the stress and confusion surrounding an acute illness or trauma may lead to a sense of disorientation in the patient. Reassure the elder patient continually. Part of that reassurance is establishing a firm relationship from the beginning. It is important to be polite, as most elder patients have grown up with and are used to more formal relationships with the people around them, especially health care workers. Explain who you are, and that you are there to help them, to stabilize their injuries or illness, and to transport them to the emergency department of the hospital. Always explain everything that you are doing to the elder patient. Do not assume that they know your routine, or that you can touch them without their permission. Gentle touch is an effective technique in managing the elder patient. Surprises or rough handling increases their level of stress.

Airway and Breathing

When assessing the airway of the elder patient, you must look, listen, and feel. Respiratory rate and depth, skin color, and use of accessory muscles should be noted. Rapid, shallow, ineffective respirations are always ominous and suggest imminent respiratory failure. Gray or ashen skin color and cyanotic nailbeds and lips suggest hypoxia and respiratory distress or failure. Elder patients in congestive heart failure are almost always diaphoretic, pale, and ashen, with rapid shallow respirations. As their degree of hypoxia and respiratory acidosis worsens, they become inattentive and difficult to engage in conversation. They get a glassy look in their eyes, and this usually occurs just prior to respiratory failure and cardiac arrest.

Listen to the sounds of the respirations. Is the patient wheezing? Are rales audible without your stethoscope? Does the patient have inspiratory stridor from narrowing of the upper airway? Is the patient making a snoring sound, which may be the result of their tongue falling back in the oropharynx, a situation easily corrected with a nasopharyngeal or oropharyngeal airway? Is the patient able to engage freely in conversation with you? Remember that some elder patients are aphasic or have cognitive difficulties that impair their ability to communicate. If the patient is unconscious, you may need to look, listen, and feel for the presence of breathing by putting your face near the nose and mouth to check for exhalation.

When assessing the airway of the elder patient, always consider the possibility of dentures or bridges. These sometimes become dislodged as the patient's state of consciousness decreases and may act as foreign bodies obstructing the airway. If the airway of the elder patient is compromised, if you are considering intubation, or if the dentures are loose or displaced, remove them carefully and place them in a clearly marked container. The patient should be assured that their dentures will be cared for properly, as they are quite expensive and important to patients.

Once the dentures are removed, it is important to remember that the elder patient's face may lose some of its structure. This is important when performing bag–valve mask ventilation. The rescuer should be certain that there is a good seal with the mask. This may involve holding the skin of the cheeks against the inflated portion of the mask in order to ensure a seal with ventilation. If the rescuer can hear air rushing past the mask and over the face, then a complete seal has not been achieved. Ventilation is ineffective. Reposition the mask and correct the difficulty. You may need to compress the loose skin of the cheeks and lower jaw against the outer inflated rim of the mask in order to make a seal.

In the case of the trauma patient, it is very important to check the chest wall. Is there even, symmetrical movement of both sides of the chest? Is there a flail segment of broken ribs on one side that moves in when the patient inhales while the rest of the chest wall moves out? Remember that the elder patient has limited functional reserve capacity. Their cardiorespiratory system has minimal ability to adapt to any illness or injury that decreases its function. The elder patient is much closer to cardiorespiratory arrest than the young patient in the face of any illness or injury that impairs their cardiorespiratory function. Flail chest is a traumatic condition involving fracture of three or more consecutive ribs in two or more places. A flail segment, because it moves paradoxically to the rest of the chest wall, impairs respiratory effort and the volume of respiration. It can be enough to severely compromise the respiratory status of a patient who has underlying lung disease.

Your patient may have a medical history of emphysema, chronic bronchitis, asthma, or any of a number of debilitating chronic pulmonary diseases. These diseases destroy lung tissue, decrease ventilatory capacity, and impair the patient's ability to take up oxygen and excrete carbon dioxide effectively. They may have little tolerance for additional insult to their lungs, either through illness, such as pneumonia or congestive heart failure, or injury, such as broken ribs or pulmonary contusion.

If you find that the patient is dyspneic, administer 100 percent oxygen by face mask immediately and monitor the result of this intervention. If possible, use pulse oximetry to measure the oxygen saturation of the blood, and try to maintain oxygen saturation at 95% or greater. If it appears that the patient is not responding appropriately with an increased ability to speak and a decrease in cyanosis, consider assisted ventilation with a bag–valve mask or endotracheal intubation.

Circulation

Assess circulation by feeling for peripheral and central pulses. First, check radial pulses at the wrists. If they are present, blood pressure is probably adequate. If they are not present, check femoral pulses, and then carotid pulses. Remember that the patient may have a considerable degree of arterial vascular disease. The patient may have had vascular operations on the femoral or carotid arteries that may interfere with adequate palpation of pulses. Always check pulses on both sides of the body. Pulses should be symmetric. Capillary refill may not be an accurate physical sign of adequate peripheral blood circulation in the elder patient. Capillary refill time is prolonged by poor circulation because of peripheral vascular disease and by hypothermia with vasoconstriction, both of which are commonly seen in the critically ill elder.

Elder patients with hemorrhage or hypovolemic shock may present with syncope, loss of consciousness, or change of mental status. Unrecognized gastrointestinal bleeding is common in elders presenting with syncope and is often overlooked until the clinician takes a history or sees evidence of melena (black or tarry stool) on the clothing or body. Hypovolemic or hypotensive elders with poor peripheral circulation may have mottling of the skin or *livido reticularis,* which is a lacy, purple, or dark reddish, netlike pattern on pale skin, and is a sign of severe vasoconstriction and impending shock.

If the patient has no palpable pulses, commence cardiopulmonary resuscitation with chest compressions. Control hemorrhage with direct pressure. Start two large-bore IVs with normal saline. Continue your assessment during stabilization and transport of the patient to the hospital.

Disability

Disability in the A, B, C, D, Es refers to impairment of mental status, including level of consciousness. The standard assessment tool for the level of consciousness is the mnemonic AVPU (Alert, response to Verbal stimuli, response to Painful stimuli, and Unresponsive). The Glasgow Coma Scale provides a more accurate and detailed assessment of mental status and has prognostic value as well. It is important, if possible, to obtain as much of the patient's medical history as possible. Elders may have a history of cerebrovascular disease and stroke with impairment of communication skills. It is important to know this history before making any judgments based on your examination of their response to voice or other stimuli.

It is also important for the prehospital health care provider to understand that assessment of disability is an ongoing or dynamic activity. It should be carried out on-scene several times as well as during transport to the hospital. The chronology of the patient's worsening, stable, or improving mental status should be reported in detail to the physician or nurse in the emergency department (ED). The patient with a severely compromised mental status may require ventilatory support or intubation to maintain the airway and breathing. Some patients who have had a massive stroke or intracranial hemorrhage lose their gag reflex, and therefore cannot protect their airway from aspiration should they vomit on-site or during transport. If the patient has lost their gag reflex, in accordance with local protocols or in consultation with medical control, the prehospital health care provider should consider intubation of the patient in order to protect the airway. This intubation should be carried out and, if appropriate, rapid sequence induction (RSI) should be considered to reduce the increase in intracranial pressure associated with intubation.

Expose

It is important in the elder trauma or medical patient to get a reasonable look at the patient's body to assess the degree and sites of injury, the depth and quality of respiration, the color of the skin, the presence of cyanosis, the presence of dependent edema, jugular venous distention, or abnormal skin markings or rash. This is done by carefully loosening or removing the patient's clothing with their permission, or, in the case of the severely injured patient, by cutting off any outer garments. It is especially important to preserve the dignity and modesty of the elder patient. These may seem like contradictory requirements, but with appropriate communication and respect for the patient, exposure can be achieved, an examination carried out, and proper clinical decisions made while respecting the modesty of the patient. Also remember that elders are more prone to hypothermia than are younger patients. As soon as adequate exposure is achieved, the patient must be covered with sheets or blankets to minimize heat loss. This is especially true for the elder trauma patient, in whom hypothermia can increase mortality.

FOCUSED ASSESSMENT

The focused assessment consists of a more detailed survey and includes taking the patient's vital signs, obtaining a medical history, and doing a physical examination of the entire patient. The prehospital health care provider must consistently pay attention to the A, B, C, D, Es. Any change in the patient's condition requiring critical intervention supersedes the focused assessment, which can be continued after the critical conditions are stabilized. The purpose of the focused assessment in the elder patient is to alert the prehospital practitioner to the extent of the medical illness or traumatic injury so that appropriate interventions and stabilization can be instituted. A carefully focused assessment may also predict the patient's course during transport to a receiving health care facility. The appropriate and correct information can then be relayed to the medical control physician and facilitate the provision of secondary and tertiary care in a timely and effective fashion. The goals and direction of the focused assessment in the traumatically injured elder patient differ from those of the medically ill elder patient. These differences result from the anatomy and physiology of aging, the differing effects of injury and illness on that physiology, and the response of the patient's physiology to those stresses. Traumatic injuries in elders can have subtle presentations but devastating outcomes. The practitioner carrying out the focused assessment must be a clever and careful detective.

The physiologic changes of the cardiovascular system associated with aging and the prevalence of chronic heart disease in the elderly limit their cardiovascular response to trauma. Elders have a decreased cardiac ejection fraction and stroke volume. They also have a decreased ability to increase their heart rate in response to hypovolemia and decreased cardiac output. Smaller volumes of blood loss can lead to more severe degrees of hypotension and shock than in younger patients. Moreover, many elder patients have underlying coronary artery disease, and periods of hypotension (associated with blood loss and decreased intravascular volume) can result in poor perfusion of the coronary arteries with ischemia and possible myocardial infarction.

A history or physical examination that suggests chest wall trauma should prompt the prehospital care provider to consider myocardial or pulmonary contusion. Elder patients with myocardial contusion tend to have more dysfunction of the heart muscle with poor cardiac output and an increased likelihood of dysrhythmias. Pulmonary contusion with hemorrhage into alveoli and lung tissue impairs lung function. The great vessels (i.e., aorta and superior and inferior vena cava) are more fragile in elder patients and much more susceptible to traumatic tears, dissection, and transsection. Either of these injuries can lead to severe or irreversible hemorrhage and shock.

The elder patient normally has diminished pulmonary reserve and function. Lung injuries, such as pulmonary contusions with bleeding into the lung tissue, pneumothoraces, hemothoraces, and multiple rib fractures, are poorly tolerated. These insults often lead to more severe hypoxia and decreased pulmonary function. Elder patients may require earlier assisted ventilation and intubation than younger patients. The prehospital health care worker should note the potential for these cardiac or pulmonary problems early in the focused assessment preparing for possible deterioration of the patient during transport to a health care facility. The prehospital practitioner should be ready to provide ventilatory and circulatory support at any time, and should alert the medical control physician if further intervention becomes necessary.

The practitioner carrying out a focused assessment should also be acutely aware of the potential for brain injury and cervical spine trauma. The elder patient is much more likely to develop subdural hematomas because of shrinkage or atrophy of the brain, the increasing space in the cranial cavity, and the fragility of the veins that run between the brain and the dura mater. Closed head injury, even without hemorrhage, may present in a more dramatic fashion in the elder patient with loss or clouding consciousness and change of mental status. Injury causing a minor concussion in a younger patient may lead to a major head injury for an elder patient. A closed head injury requires careful monitoring and support in the prehospital setting, as well as hospital admission at a health care facility. The prehospital health care worker should do a complete assessment of the patient's mental status during the focused assessment and continue to monitor that status frequently during stabilization and transport to the health care facility. Any changes must be reported immediately to the receiving physician.

The focused assessment requires palpation of the entire body, checking for tenderness, crepitus, or deformity as signs of underlying contusions and fractures. The elder's perception of pain may be altered. Therefore, the prehospital health care worker must consider the mechanism of injury and try to predict the site of injury, directing the exam accordingly.

Severe medical problems in the elder patient also present more subtly than in the younger patient and require a very careful focused assessment to uncover them. Cardiac ischemia may present as abdominal pain, jaw pain, shoulder pain, back pain, or may be silent. An acute abdomen with a perforated viscous may present as mild abdominal pain with very little tenderness. The patient can go into septic shock before major abdominal signs manifest themselves. Elder patients with a leaking abdominal aortic aneurysm may present with abdominal pain or back pain and very few other remarkable physical findings. Bilateral palpation of the femoral pulses is quite important because an asymmetric or diminished pulse on one side may indicate an impending vascular catastrophe.

Overwhelming infection in the elderly patient can present subtly as well. The patient may have impending urosepsis and present with a low-grade fever and some discomfort with urination. Elder patients can have altered temperature regulation, and may not develop a fever even if they have a severe infection. Do not be fooled by the absence of fever or, an even more ominous finding, hypothermia, in the face of possible widespread infection. If you suspect impending sepsis, be prepared for hypotension and shock. The patient may manifest only tachycardia (or normal sinus rhythm if the patient is taking beta blockers) and some mottling of the skin, or a decreased mental status from a baseline that must be obtained from relatives or neighbors.

The focused assessment is conducted from head to toe. The extremities, especially the lower extremities, should not be ignored. There is a lot of information that can be obtained by the prehospital health care worker from a thorough physical examination. The lower extremities may manifest unilateral edema secondary to deep vein thrombosis, or bilateral edema in the case of worsening congestive heart failure. There may be cyanosis of one lower extremity, suggesting arterial obstruction, or pulses may be diminished bilaterally, suggesting an abdominal vascular abnormality.

VITAL SIGNS

The prehospital health care worker should be aware of the implications of the four basic vital signs in the elder patient. These are blood pressure, pulse, respirations, and body temperature.

The implication of blood pressure in the elder patient can be complicated. Many elder patients have underlying hypertension, and may be receiving treatment with a variety of antihypertensive medications. The patient's usual blood pressure may be on the high side of normal or elevated, and a normal blood pressure may represent impending hypotension, intravascular depletion, or hemorrhage. The patient's antihypertensive medication may normally be associated with orthostatic changes when blood pressure is taken lying down and standing up. This may be a normal side effect of the medication and may not reflect decreased intravascular volume. The patient may be on a beta blocker, and as a result, be unable to generate the expected tachycardia in response to a decrease in intravascular volume (and impending shock). Pulse pressure, which is the difference between the systolic and diastolic pressure, is often used to reflect cardiac output. A wider pulse pressure generally reflects a better state of peripheral circulation. However, in an elder patient with severe peripheral vascular disease, the pulse pressure may be artificially widened because of the hardness of the patient's blood vessels.

Increased heart rate can suggest decreased intravascular volume, or a response to stress. Nevertheless, in the elder patient, pulse may be a poor marker of these events. The patient may not be able to increase their heart rate by much in response to decreasing intravascular volume or stress. The patient may be on beta blockers or have inherent autonomic nervous system dysfunction. The heart rate then becomes much less reliable as a marker for acute disease.

Respiratory rate is also a critical vital sign. Generally, patients who are stressed, in pain, or have underlying acidosis because of sepsis, diabetic ketoacidosis, or some other metabolic derangement have an increased respiratory rate. The elder patient may not have the physical ability to increase their respiratory rate very much above baseline because of stiffening of the chest wall secondary to arthritis, weakening of the respiratory muscles, or long-standing chronic lung disease. Therefore, in situations where their respiratory function is challenged by disease or injury, the respiratory rate may not reflect the degree of respiratory distress. Moreover, the patient may not be able to compensate for acidosis or increased oxygen requirements by increasing their respiratory rate significantly. For any given degree of illness, the elder may be more profoundly acidotic or hypoxic than the younger patient.

One of the most confusing vital signs in the elder patient is body temperature. The elder patient often does not have the capacity to mount a fever in response to bacterial or viral infection. Sometimes, in fact, they will become hypothermic, and this may be an important clue to overwhelming bacterial infection and impending shock. The elder patient is not able to control his or her body temperature as effectively as a younger patient. In the summer, the elder's thirst sensation is decreased, and they tend to drink inadequate amounts of fluid. They are not able to sweat efficiently, and therefore they can easily become hyperthermic, and develop severe heat stroke, which can be fatal. In the winter, they are not able to shiver effectively and generate body heat. Their subcutaneous layer of fat is often decreased compared with younger patients, and they tend to become hypothermic more rapidly. It is important for the prehospital health care worker to determine the temperature of the patient. If the patient is hypothermic, an appropriate warming procedure should be instituted immediately, as hypothermia is often deadly to the elder patient. If the patient is hyperthermic, then cooling procedures should be instituted. The elder patient is much more susceptible to the morbid and fatal effects of hypothermia and hyperthermia than the younger patient.

HISTORY

The importance of history taking is critical in the prehospital evaluation of the elder patient. The initial history taken on scene from relatives, friends, neighbors, and the patient themselves is often the most important clue to determining the underlying medical illness or traumatic injury. The prehospital health care provider can obtain the clearest and most accurate history at the time of the incident from the people who know that person the best. The prehospital health care provider also has the opportunity to survey and understand the environment in which the elder patient lives. The environment can provide clues to the injury or illness that the person has sustained. This is especially true in the case of falls, in which an assessment can provide information to the physician or nurse in the receiving facility that can be used later in discharge planning to improve home safety and reduce the likelihood of a future fall in the elder person's home.

The prehospital health care provider should obtain medicines or medical instruction documents that are vital both to the evaluation of the elder patient in the prehospital setting and also for the appropriate evaluation and treatment of the patient in the hospital. Information about patient's medications can rarely be obtained after work hours during the week and on weekends from the patient's primary care physician. The emergency physician and the receiving hospital then rely completely on information or medications that the prehospital provider brings to the emergency department in order to help the physician appropriately diagnose and treat the patient. The more chronic illnesses that the patient has, and the more medications he or she takes, the more important it is to give a complete and clear list of these medicines and their dosing. The prehospital health care worker is the emergency physician's eyes and ears in the field, and this concept is never as true as when the prehospital provider is assessing the elder patient prior to transport.

One case in which history is overwhelmingly important is in evaluating the elder patient for possible elder abuse. The dynamics of the caregivers and the state of the patient's environment provides tremendous clues indicating the possibility of neglect or active violent abuse of the elder patient. Often, the prehospital health care provider is the only person who has access to the kind of information that can be used at the receiving facility to begin to diagnose and investigate abuse.

STABILIZING AND TRANSPORTING ELDER PATIENTS

The elder patient provides unique problems for stabilization and transport. Standard protocols can be used in most situations with certain caveats. Elder patients with medical illness should be placed on a monitor, with at least one functional IV, and the patient should be placed on oxygen. If the patient has a history of congestive heart failure, intravenous fluid administration should be minimized unless the patient is in impending or noncardiogenic shock. It is easy in the prehospital or in-hospital setting to start two large-bore IVs with normal saline, and then become involved with other aspects of the patient's care, administering an excessive amount of fluid and causing the patient to go into congestive heart failure. If the decision is made to provide minimal intravenous fluid, any IVs should be set to keep vein open (TKO) only.

Some elder patients have emphysema or chronic obstructive pulmonary disease. Dyspnea should be treated with oxygen therapy; however, some of these patients may rely on their hypoxic drive to breathe. They live in a delicate balance. Providing excessive high-flow oxygen may decrease this drive to breathe and lead to respiratory arrest. If available, continuous pulse oximetry should be monitored in the elder patient. It is important while transporting patients with a history of lung disease to determine the appropriate oxygen administration with the medical control physician at the receiving hospital.

Traumatically injured elder patients should be collared and boarded if possible. Many elder patients may have moderate to severe kyphosis (forward curvature) of the spine that makes the use of conventional immobilization equipment and technique difficult. It may be necessary to provide additional padding in order to keep the patient in a stable immobilized position after a possible spine injury. Padding should also be used liberally in the elder patient who may have very little adipose (fat) tissue covering their easily bruised bony protuberances.

Elder patients with head injuries, possible intracranial hemorrhages, or strokes are at high risk for vomiting and aspiration during transport. It is very important to have suction ready and assess mental status continually. Remain aware of the possibility of vomiting and aspiration, especially when the elder is strapped to a backboard and in a cervical collar. Make sure that the elder patient is securely immobilized so that he or she can be turned to the side to help clear the airway. Perform repeated neurologic exams in order to predict which elders may require ventilatory support and intubation during a prolonged transport. Any elder patient who does not have a gag reflex is at high risk for vomiting and aspiration, and therefore communication with the medical control physician should include the possibility of intubation to protect the airway.

The prehospital health care worker should remain vigilant and aware that multiple medical problems in elder patients may interact and become additive in the situation of acute illness or injury. These patients should be monitored carefully during transport. Preparations for more intensive critical care or advanced life support interventions should be made readily available. The patient's mental status and vital signs must be checked frequently. Prepare for deterioration in the patient's condition. Once the patient becomes severely hypoxic or acidotic, the cardiac and pulmonary reserve disappear quickly leading to a respiratory arrest that may be difficult or impossible to resolve.

CONCLUSIONS

The prehospital assessment of the seriously ill or critically injured elder patient is complex and delicate, and requires all the skills and subtlety of the prehospital health care provider. Elders are different from younger persons because all of the body's organ systems are changed by aging. These changes have major implications for the prehospital provider. Even the psychosocial interaction that prehospital providers have with elders is different, as they frequently have impairments of the sensory system because of aging, and may have difficulty with vision or be hard of hearing. Those with hearing aids may be overwhelmed with sound, as those devices tend to increase all noise, not just what is being communicated to the patient. Elder patients may also have low self-esteem because of the normal aspects of aging, such as skin changes and thinning of hair. All of these differences must be kept in mind when caring for an elder patient.

Skipping any part of the initial or focused assessment or inattention to the details of the history and the environment may result in the prehospital health care provider missing important clues to illness or injury. The patient may receive inappropriate stabilization and initial treatment with increased morbidity or fatal decompensation of the patient en route to the hospital. The prehospital health care provider is responsible for the first impression of the patient that is conveyed to ED personnel. An impression formed by skilled history taking and physical examination can be life saving to the patient. False information will send ED staff down a wrong diagnostic or therapeutic road, wasting precious time. The complex chronic diseases and decreased functional capacity of the elder patient provide very little room for error. The role of the prehospital health care worker is critical both in stabilizing and transporting the patient to a receiving health care facility and in initiating proper care that will be continued in the hospital to assure speedy diagnosis, treatment, and recovery.

REVIEW QUESTIONS

Designate the following as true or false and explain your answer.

1. All septic elders present with fever.

2. All elders with suspected spinal injuries should have standard spinal immobilization.

3. Prolonged capillary refill is a sign of impending hemorrhagic shock in the injured elder patient.

4. Tachycardia is a reliable sign of hypovolemia in the elder patient.

5. Information about the elder patient's living environment is important to convey to the ED staff, especially in the case of traumatic injuries.

SUGGESTED READING

Bledsoe, B. E., R. S. Porter, and B. R. Shade, eds. 1997. *Paramedic Emergency Care*. 3d ed. Brady, Upper Saddle River, N.J.: Prentice Hall.

Caroline, N. L., ed. 1991. *Emergency Care in the Streets*. 4th ed. Boston: Little, Brown & Co.

Hafen, B. Q., K. J. Karren, and J. J. Mistovich, eds. 1996. *Prehospital Emergency Care*. 5th ed. Upper Saddle River, N.J.: Brady, Prentice Hall.

Harwood-Nuss, A., ed. 1996. *The Clinical Practice of Emergency Medicine*. 2d ed. Philadelphia: Lippincott-Raven.

Saunders, A. B., ed. 1996. *Emergency Care of the Elder Person*. St. Louis: Cracom Publications.

SECTION II

Medical Emergencies

3

Cardiovascular Disorders

Kevin A. Osgood, MD

OBJECTIVES

By the end of this chapter, the prehospital health care provider should be able to:

1 Name several symptoms of cardiovascular disease in the elder patient that would prompt activation of the EMS system.

2 Describe changes in the cardiovascular function that occur with aging.

3 Calculate the expected maximal heart rate for an 80-year-old man.

4 Name three life-threatening causes of nontraumatic chest pain in elders.

5 Identify three symptoms other than chest discomfort associated with acute myocardial infarction (heart attack) in elders.

6 Describe the prehospital treatment of the elder patient with a potentially serious cause of chest pain.

7 List three serious causes of dyspnea in elders.

8 Describe how to differentiate the causes of dyspnea in elders based on history and physical exam.

9 Describe the prehospital treatment of the elder patient with dyspnea.

10 Describe in broad terms the initial management of the elder patient who has fallen.

11 Describe the changes in cardiovascular system that lead to syncope.

12 Describe how the history and physical of an elder patient with syncope differs from that of an elder patient with a seizure.

13 Name the most common (and most lethal) tachyarrhythmia that causes syncope in elder patients.

14 Discuss the prehospital treatment of the elder patient with syncope.

Diseases of the cardiovascular system are the leading cause of death in the United States. According to the Centers for Disease Control and Prevention, nearly 32 percent of deaths in 1996 occurred as a result of heart disease, compared to 23 percent from cancer and 7 percent from stroke. The percentage of deaths caused by heart disease is even higher in the population more than 65 years of age. Cardiovascular disorders can present in a variety of ways, including cardiac arrest, chest pain, dyspnea, or syncope. These symptoms are often severe enough that the patient or their family contacts the local EMS system. The prehospital medical care provider must be aware that these symptoms in an elder person are very likely a result of a cardiovascular disorder, be familiar with the common cardiovascular disorders, and be prepared to implement life-saving therapy.

CASE

You respond to an emergency call for a man complaining of shortness of breath. On arrival, you find an elderly man with labored breathing sitting upright in a chair. He is able to tell you that he has "heart trouble" and that he began to have difficulty breathing one-half hour ago. He denies chest pain. On examination, his blood pressure is 180/90, heart rate is 130, and respiratory rate is 32. He is diaphoretic, and jugular venous distension (JVD) is present. His heart sounds are irregular, tachycardic, and without murmurs. He has mild edema in his lower extremities. His neurological examination is normal. What do you think is the problem with this man? What additional questions should you ask him? How hard is his cardiovascular system working to overcome his problem? Is he in danger? What additional treatment can you offer him? Are there any medications you should consider giving him? If so, what are the appropriate dosages?

CHANGES IN THE CARDIOVASCULAR SYSTEM WITH AGE

The function of the cardiovascular system, even in the absence of disease, declines progressively with age. It is no surprise that elders do not tolerate cardiovascular dysfunction (be it an arrhythmia or reduction in pump function) as well as younger patients. It is also more difficult for an elder person's cardiovascular system to adapt to other stresses, such as infection, gastrointestinal bleeding, or emphysema. The increasing risk of developing cardiovascular disease with aging, in combination with the expected decline in cardiovascular function, explains why elders frequently require medical care for disorders of the cardiovascular system.

With advancing age, the heart changes anatomically as the heart muscle becomes more rigid. In patients with a long history of hypertension, the muscular wall of the left ventricle increases in thickness (left ventricular hypertrophy), which also causes a marked increase in rigidity or stiffness. A rigid heart muscle is less able to increase stroke volume (the amount of blood ejected from the heart with one contraction of the ventricle) in response to the metabolic demands of the body for an increased cardiac output. In addition, a thick and rigid heart muscle has more difficulty supplying blood to the coronary arteries, and places patients at an increased risk of myocardial infarction.

In addition to anatomic changes that occur in the heart, biochemical changes within the myocardial cells lead to a decline in electrical (conduction) and muscular properties of cardiac tissue. The decline in maximum heart rate heart rate can be approximated by the following equations:

For men: Maximum heart rate = 230 − age (in years)

For women: Maximum heart rate = 225 − age (in years)

When an 80-year-old man (Max HR of 150) has a heart rate of 120, he is at 80 percent of his maximum rate. (A 30-year-old man with a heart rate of 120 is at 60 percent of his maximum rate.) The maximum heart rate attainable in elders may be further limited by the use of digoxin or antihypertensive medications such as beta blockers or calcium channel blockers.

The inability of the older heart to achieve rapid heart rates is clinically important. When looking for subtle changes in vital signs to suggest hemodynamic instability, do not wait for a fast heart rate to trigger suspicion. For example, in an elder trauma patient, major internal bleeding may be present with a heart rate of 100–110 beats per minute (bpm). Furthermore, the elder heart has limited capacity to increase cardiac output by increasing the heart rate, so it is less able to adapt to shock.

With advancing age, the electrical conduction system of the heart undergoes degenerative changes. Over time, the sinus node has fewer pacemaker cells. The His–Purkinje system undergoes fibrosis (scarring), and these changes may lead to sinus node failure or heart block, which may require placement of a permanent cardiac pacemaker.

Degeneration of the atrial and ventricular conduction pathways helps explain why elders, even in the absence of cardiac disease, are more likely than younger patients to have dysrhythmias or conduction abnormalities. Atrial fibrillation, premature ventricular contractions (PVCs), intraventricular conduction delay (widening of the QRS complex), or AV-nodal (first-, second-, or third-degree) heart block are commonly encountered in cardiac monitoring of elders. When an area of an older heart becomes ischemic from coronary artery disease, the likelihood of developing a dysrhythmia is even greater. Dysrhythmias are often poorly tolerated in elder patients.

Some dysrhythmias are well tolerated in elders and should not be concerning to the prehospital provider. As many as 80 percent of healthy elders have PVCs when their cardiac rhythm is monitored over a 24-hour period. The presence of PVCs alone should not cause concern. In the absence of signs and symptoms to suggest myocardial dysfunction or ischemia, the use of lidocaine or other antiarrhythmic for PVCs is not necessary. Underlying causes for the dysrhythmia, such as hypoxemia, acidosis, or drug effect, should be sought and corrected. If an antiarrhythmic is used, a reduced dose of the medication may be required to prevent toxicity, which occurs readily in the elderly.

With age, anatomic and functional changes also occur in blood vessels. Arterial walls lose elasticity and become less flexible. Although this occurs normally with aging, the process accelerates in the presence of atherosclerosis. Rigid arteries place a greater strain on the heart (increased afterload), and increase the risk of developing wall disruptions, such as aortic dissection or aortic aneurysm.

ASSESSING THE ELDER PATIENT FOR CARDIOVASCULAR DISEASE

Because there is a high incidence of cardiovascular disease in elders, the prehospital provider should assume that these patients have some degree of cardiovascular compromise. The EMS system is commonly activated for one of three emergency cardiovascular symptoms: Chest discomfort, Dyspnea, or Syncope.

Chest Pain

In elders, the most common causes of chest pain are myocardial infarction, aortic dissection, and pulmonary embolism.

Myocardial infarction. Elders with angina or a myocardial infarction are actually less likely to have chest pain than younger patients with these problems. Substernal chest pressure radiating to the left arm or neck, with associated diaphoresis and shortness of breath is easily recognized as a possible heart attack. However, only 60 percent of patients more than 65 years old will have classic chest discomfort with angina or myocardial infarction. In patients older than 85, the likelihood of having chest discomfort during a heart attack decreases to 40 percent. In fact, the very old (more than 85 years old) are unlikely to have chest discomfort with an acute myocardial infarction. Symptoms and signs other than chest discomfort that should prompt the prehospital health care provider to suspect angina or infarction include dyspnea, syncope, weakness, new-onset confusion, diaphoresis, nausea, and vomiting.

Do not use closed questions that require only a yes or no answer when asking an elder patient if he or she has chest discomfort. Many patients who are having a real heart attack insist that they are not having pain, but rather a "pressure," an "ache," or a "discomfort." Question the patient directly as to whether they are having any sensation in their chest that is different from normal. If discomfort is perceived, it may be anywhere between the level of the chin and the umbilicus, front or back, and in either upper extremity.

Aortic dissection. Another serious cause of chest pain in elders is aortic dissection. The wall of the aorta is composed of three layers of tissue. From inside to outside they are the *tunica intima, tunica media,* and *tunica adventitia.* Aortic dissection occurs when the innermost layer of the aorta, the intima, is torn away or eroded from the media. This usually happens to the thoracic aorta in the region known as the *aortic arch.* In this portion of the aorta, the blood has just been ejected from the heart and must make a sharp turn before flowing to the abdomen and lower extremities. There are three main branches that come off the aortic arch: the *innominate artery* (which divides into the right subclavian artery and right carotid artery), the *left carotid artery,* and the *left subclavian artery.*

The exact cause of aortic dissection is unknown. Turbulent blood flow, which occurs as the blood is sent in many different directions in the aortic arch, is thought to contribute to the disruption of the intima. In addition, patients with known hypertension are at greater risk of developing aortic dissection.

Patients at risk for aortic dissection are in the same age category as patients at risk for coronary artery disease and heart attack; therefore, any elder is at risk. The pain of aortic dissection is classically described as sudden onset; severe; and sharp, tearing, or burning in nature. The pain may be located in either the anterior or posterior chest, depending on the location of the dissection, and may change location as the tear of the inner lining of the aorta extends down the aorta.

Aortic dissection can also cause occlusion of any of the arteries that branch off the aorta, and even the aorta itself can become occluded as a result of the dissection. This happens because as the aorta dissects, the intimal flap (the part of the intima that has separated from the rest of the aorta) can occlude arteries as they branch off the aorta, and if the flap is large enough, it can occlude the entire aorta. Blood clots can also form at the point of dissection, and if they break off and become emboli, they can block smaller arteries anywhere downstream from the point of dissection. If the arterial occlusion is in the brain, it can cause a stroke or loss of consciousness. If the arterial occlusion is in an extremity, the patient may have classic symptoms of peripheral arterial occlusion: pain, pulselessness, pallor, paresthesias, and paralysis in that extremity. The prehospital provider should check for two common signs when aortic dissection is suspected. First, check for asymmetric pulses in the upper extremities. Second, check for differential blood pressures in the upper extremities. A significant differential blood pressure is a difference of more than 10 mm/Hg in the systolic pressure in the upper extremities. Abdominal pain may occur either as the lead point of the tear extends into the abdominal aorta, or as a result of the occlusion of the arteries that branch off the aorta and supply the intestines. Occlusion of the spinal arteries as they come off the descending aorta may lead to bilateral lower extremity paralysis. In addition, progressive aortic dissection may cause a loss of circulation in the lower extremities.

Aortic aneurysm is a disease of elder people different than aortic dissection. In aortic aneurysm, all three layers of the aorta become stretched and thinned. This is a painless condition that develops over a number of years. When the wall becomes so thin that the inner layers begin to tear, the aneurysm begins to cause pain. Aneurysms can occur in the thoracic or the abdominal aorta. Abdominal aortic aneurysms are sometimes palpable in the epigastrium. Thoracic aneurysms are frequently detected on chest x-rays done for other reasons. Small aneurysms rarely rupture, and are often monitored over a patient's lifetime for progression. Larger aneurysms may require immediate surgery to prevent rupture. A ruptured aneurysm usually requires emergency surgery to prevent mortality.

Aortic injury can occur from trauma. Aortic disruption from trauma is a separate entity from aortic dissection or aneurysm. It should be considered in any case where a patient is in a high-speed motor vehicle accident with a sudden deceleration, such as head-on collisions between high-speed vehicles or between a vehicle and a fixed object. The diagnosis begins in the prehospital setting with careful observation and scene assessment by the prehospital care provider.

Pulmonary embolism. Pulmonary embolism (PE) is a common cause of chest pain and can occur in both young and older patients. The mortality rate from a PE is less than 5 percent in young patients, but 15–20 percent in elders. The most common source of PE is a blood clot that forms in the leg, thigh, or pelvic veins, which is called a *deep venous thrombosis* (DVT). When a DVT becomes dislodged and travels through the venous system to the right side of the heart and then the lungs, it is called a PE. Risk factors for development of DVT and PE are the same. They include slowing of the blood in the veins (venous stasis), damage to the lining of the veins, and having blood that is more likely to clot (hypercoagulability). The patient with a prior history of DVT or PE is at significant risk for recurrent DVT or PE.

The elder population suffers the highest risk for DVT as a result of slowing of the blood. Inactivity leads to a decrease in venous return of blood from the lower extremities, and as the rate of blood flow decreases, it is more likely to clot. Although elders are often less active than younger people, inactivity (and venous stasis) is inevitable when they become sick for any reason. One injury that puts these patients at greatest risk is hip fracture. The blood is hypercoagulable (in response to clot formation around broken bone). The surrounding veins in the thigh may be injured (as a result of bony instability), and venous stasis is present because the patient cannot get up and move about to propel the blood from the legs and thighs back to the heart. One reason that early surgical fixation of hip fractures is necessary, even in the very old and frail, is to decrease the likelihood of developing DVT and PE.

The chest pain associated with PE is classically unilateral, is worse with inspiration, and is associated with some degree of dyspnea. Unfortunately, dyspnea occurs in only 80 percent of patients and chest pain in 70 percent with PE. Physical exam findings are rather nonspecific, and include tachypnea in 90 percent of cases and tachycardia in 50 percent. Only one-third of patients with PE have findings on physical exam suggestive of DVT, including calf pain, swelling, and redness.

Prehospital Management of the Elder Patient with Chest Discomfort

The principles of management of chest discomfort do not differ between the elder population and younger patients. It is important to have a high index of suspicion for serious disease. The elder patient with chest discomfort should immediately be put on a monitor, given high-flow oxygen, and have intravenous (IV) access established. Time should not be spent taking an exhaustive history at the scene once significant suspicion for cardiovascular disease has been established. The patient can be questioned about risk factors for coronary artery disease (smoking, hypertension, diabetes, and high cholesterol), but as stated previously, all elder patients are at significant risk for debilitating cardiovascular disease.

Some EMS systems have protocols that provide enough medical direction for a short transport to the hospital. Frequent reassessment of vital signs and ongoing evaluation of the cardiac rhythm on the electrocardiogram (EKG) monitor are important in all elders with chest discomfort.

Myocardial ischemia or infarction. If the discomfort is assumed to be from myocardial ischemia or infarction, sublingual nitroglycerin is the medication of first choice. Be aware, however, that elders are more likely than younger patients to become profoundly hypotensive with nitroglycerin. Nitroglycerin causes veins to dilate and pool blood. A normal response to this would be to increase the cardiac output by increasing heart rate and stroke volume, but because the elder heart cannot do this as effectively as the younger heart, the blood pressure drops more dramatically. Morphine sulfate may be useful for acute chest discomfort that is not relieved by nitroglycerin, but elders are extremely sensitive to this medication; start with a low dose of 1–2 mg IV and give additional doses if needed. Constant monitoring of a patient's vital signs is necessary to detect hypotension and poor respiratory effort. Morphine may also profoundly depress an elder patient's mental status, and should be given only under the direction of the medical control physician.

Lidocaine is used to suppress frequent premature ventricular contractions (PVCs) in patients with symptoms of cardiac ischemia. Elders metabolize this drug more slowly, and because they have a reduced total-body water content, they develop a higher blood concentration of the drug when given the same dose per kilogram as a younger person. It is advisable (except in cardiac arrest) to utilize a 1 mg/kg bolus (instead of 1.5 mg/kg) and a 1–2 mg/min IV drip (instead of 2–4 mg/min). If significant ventricular ectopy persists, a repeat dose of 0.5 mg/kg may be given every 5–10 min to a maximum total dose of 3 mg/kg.

Aspirin should also be given to all elder patients assumed to have myocardial ischemia unless they have an allergy to aspirin or cannot take medication by mouth. If possible, give 1–4 baby aspirin (depending on local protocols) to the patient to chew and then swallow. Aspirin has been shown to improve the outcome of patients with myocardial infarction when given as soon as possible after symptoms begin, so it is important that it be given in the prehospital setting for suspected myocardial ischemia or infarction.

Thrombolytic therapy is not part of routine care of the elder patient with suspected myocardial infarction in the prehospital setting. Although some out-of-hospital trials of thrombolytic medications have been performed, the benefit and safety of these medications in the prehospital setting has not yet been determined.

Aortic dissection. Treating the chest pain of aortic dissection in the same fashion as a myocardial infarction in the prehospital setting should not cause an adverse outcome. However, the use of aspirin is not recommended in the prehospital setting if aortic dissection is suspected. Hemodynamically stable patients with aortic dissection will be given additional medications on arrival in the emergency department. The goal of medical treatment is to lower the force of cardiac contraction against the dissection and lower the arterial resistance beyond the dissection (afterload). This helps reduce the shearing forces placed on the intimal tear in the aortic wall and ultimately helps prevent further dissection. The prehospital use of sublingual nitroglycerin and morphine are helpful in this situation. Once in the hospital, medications such as a beta blockers or nitroprusside are usually given intravenously for aortic dissection. Depending on the location of the intimal tear, surgery may be required to repair the aorta.

Pulmonary embolism. Oxygen is helpful to the patient with PE and is definitely indicated. If the prehospital provider feels that the chest pain is from PE, nitroglycerin is contraindicated. The reduction in right ventricular filling that occurs with nitroglycerin could lead to hypotension in the patient with PE. Pulse oximetry, if available, should be carefully monitored in patients with suspected PE. Analgesics, such as morphine, may be helpful in controlling the pain from PE, but as stated previously, vital signs and mental status should be monitored constantly. Morphine should be given only under direction of the medical control physician. Once the patient arrives at the hospital, anticoagulation with heparin can be initiated, the diagnosis of PE can be confirmed with radiologic testing, and thrombolytic therapy may be given.

Dyspnea. The patient in our case is presenting with dyspnea. *Dyspnea* is difficulty breathing as perceived by the patient. This rather frightening symptom has a wide range of causes. In elders it is frequently a symptom of pulmonary or cardiovascular disease. The sensation of dyspnea is present whenever very small changes in oxygen concentration are detected in the arterial blood supply by specialized structures called the *carotid* and *aortic bodies*. Dyspnea may be associated with other symptoms that result from other cardiovascular problems, such as dyspnea associated with fever, chills, and cough with discolored phlegm in the patient with pneumonia.

Dyspnea is commonly associated with myocardial infarction, PE, and a variety of other lung diseases, including chronic obstructive pulmonary disease. Dyspnea is frequently a primary sign of congestive heart failure in elders.

RETURNING TO THE CASE

Clearly, the man in our case is presenting with congestive heart failure (CHF). He has a history of "heart trouble" and complains of the acute onset of dyspnea. He is tachycardic and tachypneic, and mildly hypotensive. Patients with congestive heart failure are often hypertensive initially, but as their heart function gets worse and cardiac output drops, they can become hypotensive. Hypotension in CHF is a "red flag" for a critically ill patient. He is also diaphoretic and has JVD, which are also common signs of CHF. His heart sounds are irregular, suggesting that he is in atrial fibrillation. Elders depend on the "atrial kick" from normal sinus rhythm to maintain their cardiac output. New atrial fibrillation can cause CHF in an elder patient who already has heart disease. It would be important for the prehospital care provider to ask the patient or his relatives if he has had CHF before, if he has had a previous heart attack, and what medications he is currently taking. Answering these questions may provide additional clues to the diagnosis and make treatment faster and more effective. CHF is treatable, and the prehospital care provider should reassure the patient and family.

Congestive Heart Failure

The occurrence of CHF is frequent in elders and is the most common hospital discharge diagnosis in the United States in the elder population. *Congestive heart failure* is defined as a failure of the myocardium to pump adequate blood volume to meet the metabolic demands of the body. The left ventricle has the greatest workload of any of the four chambers. It is responsible for pumping blood the longest distance, and must generate the greatest force. Left ventricular failure is the primary cause of most cases of CHF.

The two most common causes of CHF are coronary artery disease and hypertension, both of which occur over a prolonged period and result in irreversible damage to the heart muscle. When the force of cardiac contraction decreases, changes occur in the body, resulting in fluid retention and increased adrenergic stimulation, which in turn augments the function of the failing heart. Eventually, the ability to maintain cardiac output fails, and the diseased heart muscle becomes progressively symptomatic.

CHF can be thought of as deterioration of the ventricular muscle that affects its ability to pump blood effectively to the systemic circulation. The stasis of blood in the left ventricle results in backup of blood into the pulmonary tree and inadequate oxygenation of the static blood flow through the left ventricle. Fluid congestion in the lungs causes impaired oxygen and carbon dioxide exchange at the alveolar membrane, resulting in the symptom of dyspnea. The patient may become dyspneic when lying supine at night (paroxysmal nocturnal dyspnea) or with activity (dyspnea on exertion). Patients with CHF may be found in severe pulmonary edema with diaphoresis, cyanosis, and a panicked appearance, gasping for breath. If possible, question the patient about prior episodes of dyspnea, as many patients with heart failure have had numerous episodes of symptomatic CHF prior to seeking medical attention. The patient should also be asked about underlying lung problems and use of inhalers. An exacerbation of chronic obstructive pulmonary disease (COPD) can appear identical to CHF in the prehospital setting. Patients with CHF or COPD exacerbations may also have chest pressure that is indistinguishable from myocardial ischemia in the prehospital setting.

Patients with CHF frequently have *rales* on physical exam, a crackling sound easily detected by auscultation. Wheezing may or may not be present in CHF. Mental status changes can occur as a result of hypoxia or hypercarbia (increased CO_2 levels) of the blood. The absence of pedal edema does not rule out the diagnosis of CHF. Vital signs are important in choosing appropriate pharmacological intervention.

Because dyspnea in elders is commonly a symptom of cardiac etiology, these patients should have early placement of cardiac monitor leads, be placed on supplemental oxygen, and have IV access established. Frequent reassessment of vital signs, cardiac rhythm, and mental status (to assess for hypoxemia) are critical elements of the patient's evaluation and management.

Local EMS protocols should be followed. Manage patients with suspected myocardial infarction or PE as described in the section on chest discomfort. Give the patient with a suspected COPD exacerbation an inhaled beta-agonist, such as albuterol, enroute to the hospital. Give patients with dyspnea supplemental oxygen, regardless of the etiology of the dyspnea.

Treatment of CHF varies depending on the severity of illness and the patient's vital signs. The treatment begins with supplemental oxygen and, if indicated, assisted ventilation with a bag-valve mask. Patients require ventilatory assistance if the respiratory rate is less than 10 or greater than 24 breaths per min. Once this is accomplished, direct attention at decreasing venous return to the left heart and reducing the load against which the heart is pumping (afterload). If the patient has CHF, administer sublingual nitroglycerin if the systolic blood pressure is greater than 110 mmHg. Nitroglycerin dilates the venous system, decreasing return of blood to the right heart, lungs, and left heart (preload). It also decreases systolic blood pressure, thus reducing afterload.

Furosemide (Lasix®) has a rapid effect by acting as a vasodilator and decreasing preload, and then a slower diuretic effect that also decreases preload and can continue for up to 6 hours. Give 20–80 mg IV or IM if IV access cannot be established. If a patient is already on furosemide, use their current dose as a guide. In acute CHF, a reasonable rule of thumb is to give the same number of milligrams IV as the patient takes orally per dose. Lower initial doses are advised in elders who have never had furosemide previously. Extreme caution should be used if the patient's systolic blood pressure is below 100 mmHg. Follow local protocols and the guidance of medical control.

Although furosemide is the most commonly used loop diuretic in the prehospital setting, bumetanide (Bumex®) is also used. The dose of bumetanide ranges from 0.5 mg to 2 mg IV, and 1 mg of bumetanide is approximately equal to 40 mg of furosemide. Again, if a patient is already on bumetanide, use their usual dose as a guide, and observe carefully for hypotension. Always remember that even if a patient is on a high dose of furosemide, they may respond to a lower equivalent dose of bumetanide, especially if they have never had bumetanide in the past.

Morphine is occasionally used in the prehospital setting in the management of CHF. It is a vasodilator (reducing preload) and an anxiolytic, which may help make a frightened patient more comfortable during respiratory distress. However, IV morphine is both a central nervous system and a respiratory depressant, and its effects are more pronounced in elders. As a result of IV morphine use, an elder patient in CHF may need intubation for airway control because of these side effects. The use of morphine in the management of CHF in elders is not routine, and should be done only under the direction of the medical control physician.

Other medications that may be used to treat CHF that are occasionally used in the prehospital setting or during hospital-to-hospital transfers include the following:

Dobutamine, 2–20 µg/kg/min IV
Dopamine, 5–15 µg/kg/min IV
Norepinephrine, 0.5–30 µg/min IV

These agents have specific indications and are used only when the patient is in shock. They should be given only under the direction of the medical control physician.

In addition, when the patient is in CHF and has a normal blood pressure or is hypertensive, the following medications may occasionally be indicated:

Nitroglycerin, 10–20 µg/min IV for decreasing preload and afterload
Nitroprusside, 0.1–5.0 µg/kg/min IV for decreasing afterload

If these medications, in tandem with ventilator support, do not relieve the symptoms of CHF, patients may require emergency coronary artery angiography to assess whether improvement in coronary perfusion can be achieved to improve cardiac pump function.

Although the treatment of severe CHF requires aggressive management in the prehospital environment, mild CHF may respond to furosemide and oxygen therapy. For patients with mild symptoms, a greater amount of time can be spent taking a history and performing a physical exam as the EMS unit transports the patient to the hospital. Without chest x-rays and other testing in the prehospital setting, there is a significant percentage of patients whose cause of dyspnea will be undiagnosed at the time of arrival at the emergency department. If the diagnosis is known, initiate therapy per local EMS protocol. Otherwise, stabilize and transport the patient to the hospital, where more definitive testing and treatment can be performed.

Syncope

Syncope can be defined as a brief loss of consciousness (LOC) resulting from hypoperfusion of the brain. Syncope is not caused by head trauma or seizure. In a patient found down, it may be impossible to determine whether a fall with head injury caused the LOC (concussion) or a syncopal event caused the LOC with a subsequent fall and head injury. For any elder with a fall, try to determine the cause of the fall in addition to screening the patient for injury. Always consider syncope as a primary cause of LOC or trauma.

Patients with syncope usually return to their normal neurologic state within 1 min of the event. With seizures, abnormal states of consciousness may persist. The patient who is not fully conscious after EMS arrival should be evaluated for hypoglycemia, hypoxemia, or drug overdose.

Syncope can be caused by central nervous system (CNS) dysfunction, autonomic nervous system irregularity (neurocardiogenic syncope), cardiac dysfunction, or orthostatic hypotension. Often in elders, several factors may contribute to the syncope at once. Occasionally, younger patients with psychiatric disorders behave as if they are unconscious or unresponsive, but this type of behavior is extremely rare in the elder patient.

Central Nervous System Dysfunction

In syncope, there must be disruption of neuronal function in both left and right cerebral hemispheres simultaneously or disruption of function in the brainstem. Vertebrobasilar insufficiency (VBI) is a transient ischemic attack of the brainstem. The vertebral arteries (not the carotid arteries) usually provide the blood supply to the brainstem. The vertebral arteries unite intracranially to form the basilar artery, which then gives off branches to the brainstem. Patients with VBI may experience dizziness prior to the syncopal event. VBI may also occur with certain neck movements if the vertebral arteries are compressed along their path within the vertebral column. Patients with VBI are usually placed on a daily dose of aspirin after the diagnosis is confirmed.

Intracranial hemorrhage can result in a brief loss of consciousness. However, unlike patients with syncope, these patients may fail to return to normal neurologic status. If they regain consciousness, they frequently complain of a headache. Patients with intracranial hemorrhage may require surgery to stop the bleeding or prevent further bleeding.

Neurocardiogenic Syncope

Neurocardiogenic syncope is the most common type of syncope in both younger and elder patients. Neurocardiogenic syncope (also called *fainting, vasovagal syncope,* or *vasodepressor syncope*) results from autonomic nervous system irregularity. Stimulation of the parasympathetic nervous system and suppression of the sympathetic nervous system causes a drop in blood pressure and heart rate, resulting in decreased cardiac output, poor brain perfusion, and unconsciousness. Neurocardiogenic syncope can be associated with extreme fear, emotional stress, or pain in susceptible individuals (e.g., passing out when blood is drawn). This type of syncope can also occur in elders after urinating (micturition syncope), with bowel movements accompanied by straining (defecation syncope), or during a severe coughing spell (tussive syncope). Nausea, diaphoresis, and tunnel vision usually precede the fainting spell; however, elders may not describe these symptoms clearly. The management of neurocardiogenic syncope consists of assessment for injury (if the patient fell) with appropriate stabilization, and a search for other, more serious causes of syncope. Provide supplemental oxygen, initiate cardiac monitoring, and establish IV access in the prehospital environment.

Cardiac Syncope

In the elder patient, cardiac dysfunction is the most common cause of syncope. In cardiac syncope, inadequate perfusion of the brain results from cardiac pump dysfunction. Unlike patients with vasovagal syncope, patients with cardiac syncope typically feel well and have no warning prior to their loss of consciousness. The syncopal event can occur at rest or with exertion. A return to consciousness occurs when the cardiac output returns to the level required by the brain to maintain alertness. The decrease in cardiac output may be from an electrical (conduction) problem, a mechanical (muscular) problem, or a combination of both.

Electrical problems are the most common cause of cardiac syncope. Recall that cardiac output is the product of stroke volume and heart rate (CO = SV × HR). When the heart rate decreases, the stroke volume must increase to maintain cardiac output. In syncope caused by bradycardia, stroke volume cannot increase enough to maintain cardiac output. The flow of blood to the brain decreases and the patient becomes unconscious. The aging heart becomes more rigid, cannot expand to accommodate increased blood return, and cannot increase stroke volume in the face of decreasing heart rate in the same manner as a younger heart. Bradycardia is poorly tolerated in elders and often causes syncope.

Sick sinus syndrome is one cause of transient, sinus bradycardia that may result in syncope. Lenegre's disease (fibrosis of the His–Purkinje bundles) can cause high-degree atrioventricular block in elders that may result in syncope. Overmedication with a beta blocker or calcium channel blocker can cause bradycardic syncope, especially in the elder patient in whom degeneration of the electrical system already exists.

When you look at the "cardiac output" equation, it would seem that the greater the heart rate, the greater the cardiac output. In reality, as heart rate becomes faster, the stroke volume begins to decline. With an increased heart rate, diastolic filling time decreases, as does diastolic volume. As the heart rate becomes very fast (somewhere more than 120–140 bpm in elders), stroke volume decreases, cardiac output declines, and loss of consciousness may occur. Because of age related anatomic changes, elders' hearts require a longer time for ventricular filling. In addition, increases in heart rate result in increases in myocardial oxygen demand. Because elders are more likely to have coronary artery disease, they may be less capable of increasing myocardial oxygen supply. This precipites ischemia and left ventricular dysfunction when heart rate increases.

Tachycardia is poorly tolerated in elders and often causes syncope in the elder population. The most common tachyarrhythmia causing syncope in elders is ventricular tachycardia. This life-threatening arrhythmia may not be sustained, and if the patient quickly returns to a normal sinus rhythm or at least a slower rhythm that allows the heart to sustain a high enough blood pressure for adequate tissue perfusion, the patient becomes conscious again. This frequently happens prior to EMS arrival, so the prehospital provider must have a high index of suspicion for a life-threatening arrhythmia in any elder patient with syncope, even if they have no complaints or abnormal physical findings at the scene. Ventricular tachycardia may also occur as a result of new-onset myocardial ischemia or long-standing cardiac structural disease. Occasionally it is the result of an electrolyte abnormality (hypokalemia), adverse effect of medications, or a drug overdose (e.g., tricyclic antidepressants, cocaine). Although the prehospital provider should consider other causes of ventricular tachycardia, always bear in mind that ventricular tachycardia in the elder age group is usually the result of an underlying cardiac problem, and should be treated accordingly.

Atrial fibrillation is the most common arrhythmia in the elder population. Although atrial fibrillation with a controlled ventricular response is well tolerated, atrial fibrillation with an *uncontrolled* or rapid ventricular response is poorly tolerated in elders and may contribute to syncope. The increased heart rate decreases ventricular filling time and stroke volume. There is also a decrease in the efficiency of ventricular filling because of the loss of a synchronous atrial pump (also called the *atrial kick*). Always consider other causes of syncope (such as pulmonary embolus, myocardial infarction, or severe infection) in the patient with rapid atrial fibrillation.

Manage cardiac syncope by treating the dysrhythmia and any underlying cause of the dysrhythmia. Early cardiac monitoring, administering supplemental oxygen, and establishing IV access are essential in elders with syncope. Initial management of the dysrhythmia and a search for an underlying cause can begin in the prehospital setting. Ultimately, such patients may require a pacemaker for bradycardia, angioplasty, coronary stents or bypass surgery for coronary artery disease, or an automatic implantable cardiac defibrillator for ventricular tachycardia. Patients who already have a pacemaker or defibrillator implanted should have their cardiac rhythm monitored to ensure the device is functioning properly. Documentation of the dysrhythmia and correlation of rhythm strip findings with symptoms is critical in managing these patients.

Cardiac syncope can also be caused by mechanical obstruction. The most common in elders is aortic stenosis. In aortic stenosis, the aortic valve outlet becomes progressively smaller. When stroke volume cannot support perfusion of the brain, syncope occurs. Syncope from aortic stenosis classically occurs with exertion. Patients regain consciousness soon after their collapse as there is usually sufficient blood flow allowed through the aortic valve to meet the oxygen needs of both the brain and the skeletal muscles in the absence of exercise. Patients with aortic stenosis severe enough to cause syncope require a valve opening procedure (valvuloplasty) or aortic valve replacement to prevent future syncopal events.

The prehospital provider should use extreme caution in giving nitroglycerin to elder patients with severe aortic stenosis (patients should be asked if they have a history of aortic stenosis) because this may cause syncope, even with small doses. Any elder patient with suspected myocardial ischemia or infarction should be carefully monitored and given nitroglycerin only under direction of the medical control physician.

Orthostatic Hypotension

Orthostatic hypotension can also cause syncope in the elder population. This occurs when there is inadequate return of venous blood to the heart (as in blood loss) or inadequate vascular constriction in the arterial circulation (as with certain medications), resulting in decreased perfusion of the brain. Elders are more likely to develop orthostatic hypotension because they have decreased intravascular volume, loss of arterial elastasticity, and increased rigidity of the heart muscle. As many as 20 percent of elders have *orthostatic hypotension*, defined as a decrease in systolic blood pressure of at least 20 mmHg, in the absence of any acute disease.

Syncope may be the chief complaint of patients with severe gastrointestinal bleeding (GI bleed) or a ruptured abdominal aortic aneurysm (AAA). A history of other symptoms in these patients can often be obtained from the patient or family members. Patients with a ruptured AAA may report back or abdominal pain before their collapse and may have a palpable pulsatile mass in their epigastrium. Patients with a severe GI bleed may have black- or burgundy-colored stools, hematemesis, and conjunctival pallor from anemia. Patients should be asked about the use of blood pressure medication and diuretics because these medicines contribute to syncope in elders. Patients with orthostatic hypotension usually have tachycardia. However, the tachycardic response in elders may not be as great as in younger patients, especially if they are taking beta blockers.

Prehospital Management of the Geriatric Patient with Syncope

There are many causes of syncope in elders and a diagnosis is not always readily apparent in the prehospital environment. The chief complaint may be a fall, an injury from a fall, or a loss of consciousness. Falls are the leading cause of injury in the elderly. Many elderly patients say they lost their balance or tripped to explain the cause of their fall. All of these patients should be screened for syncope as well as any injuries that they sustained.

Early provision of supplemental oxygen, initiation of cardiac monitoring, and establishing IV access in the prehospital environment allows diagnosis and treatment of lethal cardiac dysrhythmias. The history of events prior to the loss of consciousness and findings on physical exam may be key to establishing the etiology of a syncopal event. If a reason for the syncope is determined, then the prehospital health care provider can select and initiate appropriate treatment. All elder patients with syncope should be closely monitored and transferred to the nearest emergency department for further evaluation and management.

SUMMARY

Elders are more likely to have cardiovascular disease than younger patients. They may present with chest discomfort, dyspnea, syncope, or other less severe symptoms. Awareness of the changes that occur in the cardiovascular system with aging and of the manner in which cardiovascular disease manifests in elders should help prepare the prehospital health care provider to manage the medical problems of our aging population.

REVIEW QUESTIONS

1. Which disease is the leading cause of death for elder Americans?
   a. Stroke
   b. Heart disease
   c. Cancer
   d. Trauma

2. All of the following changes occur in the heart with aging *except*
   a. the heart muscle becomes more rigid
   b. it is harder to increase stroke volume in response to increased metabolic demand
   c. coronary arteries become larger and easier to perfuse
   d. it is harder to increase cardiac output

3. What is the maximum predicted heart rate (beats per minute) of an 85-year-old man?
   a. 145 bpm
   b. 185 bpm
   c. 140 bpm
   d. 230 bpm

4. Elder persons are more likely to have cardiac dysrhythmias because of changes in the
   a. muscular tissue of the heart
   b. electrical conduction system of the heart
   c. walls of the coronary arteries
   d. heart valves

5. All of the following are cardiovascular symptoms in the elderly *except*
   a. chest pain
   b. dyspnea
   c. syncope
   d. left arm weakness

6. A patient with aortic dissection
   a. will describe slow onset of pressure-like chest pain radiating down the left arm
   b. will describe sudden onset of severe burning or tearing chest pain radiating to the back

    c. is not likely to have blood clots form at the site of dissection

    d. does not have coronary artery disease

7. All of the following are risk factors for coronary artery disease *except*
   a. emphysema
   b. hypertension
   c. smoking
   d. high cholesterol

8. When giving lidocaine to an elder patient, it is important to remember that
   a. lidocaine is metabolized more slowly than in younger patients
   b. the dosage given is the same as for younger patients
   c. lidocaine should be given to all patients with suspected ischemia
   d. elder patients do not get seizures from lidocaine toxicity

9. Elder patients with chest pain suspected to be cardiac in origin
   a. should swallow 4 coated aspirin as soon as possible after EMS arrival
   b. should chew 1–4 baby aspirin as soon as possible after EMS arrival
   c. should chew 1–4 baby aspirin as soon as possible unless they have an aspirin allergy
   d. should be given 4 aspirin by mouth even if they are unable to swallow

10. The most common tachyarrhythmia to cause syncope in elders is
    a. sinus tachycardia
    b. rapid atrial fibrillation
    c. supraventricular tachycardia (SVT)
    d. ventricular tachycardia

11. When evaluating and treating an elder patient with syncope, the pre-hospital provider should
    a. administer supplemental oxygen
    b. place the patient on a cardiac monitor
    c. never place the patient in a collar and on a backboard
    d. establish IV access

SUGGESTED READING

Abrams, W. B., M. H. Beers, and R. Berkow. 1995. The Merck manual of geriatrics, 2d ed., Merck Research Laboratories.

Albrich, J. M. 1997. Congestive heart failure: A state-of-the-art review of clinical pitfalls, evaluation strategies, and recent advances in drug therapy. *Emergency Medicine Reports* 18(16–17).

Aronow, W. S. and D. D. Tresch, eds. 1996. Coronary artery disease in the elderly. *Clinics in Geriatric Medicine* 12(1).

Colucciello, S. A. 1996. Pulmonary embolism: A rational approach to the patient with suspected PE. *Emergency Medicine Reports* 17(12–13).

Henderson, M. C. and S. D. Prabhu, 1997. Syncope: Current diagnosis and treatment. *Current Problems in Cardiology,* May.

Kiel, D. P. 1993. The evaluation of falls in the emergency department. *Clinics in Geriatric Medicine* 9(3):591–599.

Reichel, W., ed. 1995. Care of the elderly: Clinical aspects of aging, 4th ed. Williams & Wilkins.

Sanders, A. B., ed. 1996. Emergency care of the elder person, Beverly Cracom.

Zappa, M. J. 1993. Recognition and management of acute aortic dissection and thoracic aortic aneurysm. *Emergency Medicine Reports* 14(1).

4

Pulmonary Disorders

Mark Williams, MD

OBJECTIVES

By the end of this chapter, the prehospital health care provider should be able to:

1 Recognize manifestations of emphysema and asthma.

2 Discuss emergent treatment of emphysema and asthma.

3 Recognize causes of acute and subacute decompensation in chronic obstructive pulmonary disease (COPD) patients.

4 Identify risk factors for pulmonary embolus in elders.

5 Appreciate the range of symptomatic presentation in patients with pulmonary embolus (PE).

6 Recognize the manifestations of pneumonia and bronchitis in elders.

7 Recognize the significance of vital signs in patients with pneumonia.

8 Appreciate wide spectrum of supportive treatments for patients with pneumonia.

9 Recognize importance and range of supportive care in patients with pneumonia.

10 Recognize the subtlety of presentation in elder patients with pneumothorax.

11 Recognize the signs and symptoms of tension pneumothorax and appropriate treatment.

12 Distinguish between pulmonary and gastrointestinal (GI) sources of bleeding.

13 Distinguish massive from minor hemoptysis.

The respiratory system is a vital body system responsible for delivery of oxygen to body tissues as well as removal of the metabolic waste product carbon dioxide (CO_2). Respiratory emergencies in elders are one of the most common complaints prompting EMS calls. Their immediate recognition and management can be life saving. This chapter discusses special considerations of elder patients with regard to pulmonary disease and its prehospital management.

CASE

The patient is an elderly woman who is found sitting up in her bed, hunched over a night table and breathing rapidly. Her skin is very pale and her lips have a bluish color. Her fingertips have nicotine stains. She can barely speak, but the family tells you her shortness of breath has been worsening for 2 days. On physical examination, her blood pressure is 160/90, her heart rate is 110, and her respiratory rate is 30 breaths per minute. You can hear wheezing and rhonchi bilaterally, and she does not seem to be moving much air. Heart tones are distant and barely audible. She is thin and has a barrel-shaped chest. What do you think is the problem with this woman? What additional history should you ask for? How sick is she? Is she in danger? What treatment should you offer? What medications should you give, and in what dosages?

OBSTRUCTIVE LUNG DISEASE

Chronic obstructive pulmonary disease (COPD) is a common cause of shortness of breath for those over age 50 and affects an estimated 15 percent of the U.S. population. COPD is generally described as a mixture of three diseases, with the hallmark feature being airway outflow obstruction. The three conditions are emphysema (destruction and collapse of terminal airways), asthma (reversible airway reactivity), and chronic bronchitis (airway inflammation). These three conditions vary in their degree of severity in each patient with COPD, although elders are afflicted primarily with emphysema and/or chronic bronchitis. This section describes each component and discusses clinical aspects and prehospital management.

Emphysema is characterized by destruction of lung tissue that supports the alveoli (air sacs) and is commonly seen in elders after years of smoking. The gradual destruction of both lung tissue and capillaries leads to decreased area for gas exchange and increased resistance to pulmonary blood flow. Weakening of the walls of bronchioles (small airways) causes less recoil and results in air entrapment in the lungs. In a normal person, an increase in arterial carbon dioxide concentration ($PaCO_2$) stimulates repiratory drive. In the elder patient with emphysema, over time arterial oxygen concentration (PaO_2) decreases and $PaCO_2$ increases, and the patient becomes dependent on hypoxic drive to control his or her respirations. Low PaO_2 stimulates red blood cell production (polycythemia), creating the "pink puffer" appearance of these patients.

Chronic bronchitis is characterized by increased mucus production and an increased number of mucus-producing cells in the bronchial tree, resulting in mucus plugging and increased airway inflammation and resistance. Unlike emphysema, there is no alveolar destruction, and diffusion of gases remains normal in chronic bronchitis. However, gas exchange is decreased because of lowered alveolar ventilation, which ultimately leads to hypoxia and hypercarbia. These patients tend to be overweight and cyanotic, thus creating their "blue bloater" appearance. Both emphysema and chronic bronchitis can result in pulmonary hypertension and right ventricular hypertrophy. These conditions can deteriorate into cor pulmonale (right heart failure), which is ultimately fatal.

Asthma is characterized by reversible airway reactivity (bronchospasm) and may be caused by a variety of stimuli. Asthma is diagnosed as a primary condition more often in a younger patient, but can persist into older age. It is rarely a primary diagnosis in an older person.

RETURNING TO THE CASE

The woman in our case is presenting with an exacerbation of COPD. She has a long history of cigarette smoking and complains of shortness of breath. When you find her, she is sitting in the classic tripod position, leaning forward and resting her weight on both her hands. This provides her with the best use of her breathing muscles, the so-called mechanical advantage. She is wheezing, which reflects airway obstruction, and has rhonchi, because of inflammation. Many patients with COPD have worsening of their disease when they develop an upper respiratory tract infection or bronchitis. Air becomes trapped in their lungs, and they are not able to exchange the respiratory gases oxygen and carbon dioxide. Their blood oxygen gets very low, and carbon dioxide increases, making them acidotic. They experience terrible respiratory distress and air hunger. The lack of air movement in this patient suggests that she is very sick. Immediately, provide her with nebulized albuterol and oxygen. Remember that she may be a CO_2 "retainer" (explained later), and may lose her respiratory drive and stop

(continued)

breathing. You should ask the patient or the family when she was last treated in the emergency department for COPD, and whether she was hospitalized or intubated. Find out if she is on home oxygen, what medications she takes, and whether she has been compliant.

Elder patients with COPD typically present with shortness of breath as their main complaint. Other symptoms may include cough (common in those with a more predominant component of chronic bronchitis or asthma), chest pain or minor hemoptysis (expectorated blood). Some elder patients may initially have symptoms from other medical or surgical disease, but because of limited pulmonary reserve become short of breath and then call EMS. Appropriate history includes duration of symptoms, medications, medical history, history of hospitalizations, and history of intubation. Those with end-stage COPD may be dependent on oxygen or steroids and the dose of either should be noted, as well as the time the patient was last on oxygen or the time the last dose of steroid was taken. Patients short of breath with deterioration of mental status are of significant concern.

COPD is usually exacerbated by some insult to the already frail pulmonary system. Life-threatening acute decompensation can be caused by pneumothorax, pulmonary embolism (PE), or acute collapse of a segment of the lung. Other subacute causes include bronchitis, pneumonia, pulmonary compression from abdominal ascites or pleural effusion, trauma, or other neuromuscular or metabolic disease. Factors such as patient noncompliance with medications, insufficient therapy, or inappropriate therapy may also cause respiratory decompensation.

Elder patients with exacerbation of COPD are usually tachypneic, tachycardic, and may be hypertensive and appear anxious. The *tripod stance* (upright with hands on knees) and pursed lip respirations are signs of severe respiratory distress. Degree of respiratory distress is important to note, and is assessed by evaluation of accessory muscle use and the patient's pattern of speech. Broken sentences because of a need for a breath is often indicative of a serious respiratory condition. Further physical examination may reveal wheezing and/or diminished breath sounds. Some patients exhibit a barrel-shaped chest (increased anterioposterior diameter), cachexia (wasted appearance), pink skin, and clubbing of the fingernails. Others are cyanotic and obese, with jugular venous distension and ankle edema. It is important to remember that in elder patients "all that wheezes is not asthma." Other causes of wheezing include congestive heart failure, foreign body aspiration, neoplasms (lung cancer or other tumors), pulmonary embolus, toxic gas inhalation, and allergic or analphylactic reactions.

Prehospital management of COPD patients depends on the severity of symptoms. Cardiac monitoring, IV access, and continuous pulse oximetry with frequent reassessment are key in when treating and transporting these patients. Oxygen must be given, but remember that oxygen may decrease the respiratory drive in COPD patients. Although this may seem illogical, the pathophysiology of emphysema and chronic bronchitis causes a patient's respiratory effort to be driven by *hypoxia* (low oxygen levels) rather than increased CO_2 concentration (increased CO_2 concentration causes respiratory drive in patients with normal lungs). Administering 10 l by face mask and obliterating that hypoxic drive may cause respiratory arrest and worsen the problems of an already decompensated patient. Hypercarbia can ultimately cause life-threatening arrhythmias and cardiac arrest. To avoid these complications, be prepared to use a bag–valve mask to ventilate, or to intubate.

If a patient is dependent on home oxygen therapy and is having a mild COPD exacerbation, increasing their oxygen by 2 l/min by nasal cannula may be sufficient. If an elder patient with COPD exacerbation is profoundly hypoxic and a higher concentration of oxygen is required, careful monitoring of pulse oximetry and respiratory effort is mandatory. A reasonable goal would be to keep the pulse oximetry between 90 percent and 95 percent. If a patient loses his or her respiratory drive and pulse oximetry is high, the prehospital provider should assist ventilations with a bag–valve mask. Always be prepared to intubate if necessary.

Other treatment modalities are aimed at the reversible components of COPD. Inhaled beta agonists (albuterol) or anticholinergics (ipratroprium bromide) can reduce bronchospasm over a short period of time. Steroids (methylprednisolone) are included in some prehospital protocols and can reduce airway inflammation, but their effect is not immediate and usually does not occur until 6 hr after administration. As previously mentioned, mental status changes are an ominous sign that hypoxia and hypercarbia are worsening. In the event that hypoxic respiratory failure occurs, it becomes necessary to establish an airway via an endotracheal tube. Adhere to regional protocols, transport and contact medical control. Patients presenting with a predominant asthma component may be in status asthmaticus. By definition, this is an attack that is refractory to usual therapy, and the patient demonstrates a decline in mental status or develops a silent chest with little or no air movement. These patients also require a secure airway with endotracheal intubation, high flow oxygen, and rapid transport. Treatment of elder patients in status asthmaticus with epinephrine is controversial and often contraindicated because epinephrine may cause hypertension or coronary ischemia. It may be difficult to differentiate in the field if a patient's COPD is predominantly emphysema or asthma, except that emphysema is much more common in elders. The use of epinephrine in elder patients suspected of being in status asthmaticus should be done according to local protocols and under direction of the medical control physician.

PULMONARY EMBOLUS

Pulmonary embolus (PE) is a life-threatening cause of chest pain or shortness of breath and is defined as a sudden blockage of the pulmonary artery, usually by a clot transported from the venous system of the pelvis or upper thigh. Blood clots in the calf rarely embolize but may extend to the upper thigh and then embolize. PE accounts for one-third of all postoperative deaths, the incidence increases with age and it is thought to be responsible for at least 50,000 deaths per year. Pulmonary emboli are found at autopsy in as many as 40–50 percent of all patients and are believed to be the cause of death in 5–10 percent of those patients.

Risk factors for PE in elders are numerous and include history of recent and prolonged immobilization, obesity or recent MI, recent surgery (including gynecologic, thoracic, abdominal, or orthopedic), cancer, cardiopulmonary disease, history of PE or deep venous thrombosis (DVT) or current thrombophlebitis.

Patients with PE have a wide variety of presentations. The most common complaint is sudden shortness of breath with or without chest pain. Other presenting symptoms can include fatigue, syncope (passing out), apprehension, leg pain or swelling, low grade fever, and hemoptysis (expectorating blood). Physical examination can reveal tachypnea, tachycardia, wheezing on chest auscultation, irregular heart beat (atrial fibrillation), and leg or calf swelling or redness. Pulse oximetry can be alarmingly low (less than 70 percent); however, it can be normal. In cases of massive PE, jugular venous distension, hepatomegaly, and falling blood pressure may occur.

Diagnosis of PE is difficult and elusive in the elderly and may be confounded by underlying cardiopulmonary disease. Definitive testing such as radiography, nuclear medicine tests (V/Q scans), or pulmonary angiography is hospital based. Proper prehospital assessment includes presence or absence of risk factors and severity of symptoms.

Prehospital management can be as simple as transporting in position of comfort and administration of supplemental oxygen as needed. In more severely affected patients, an effective airway must be established and maintained with high flow oxygen and continuous pulse oximetry monitoring. Those with impending respiratory arrest should be intubated. In those with poor vital signs or impending circulatory collapse, establishment of intravenous access and administration of fluids may be life saving. Some patients may progress to refractory hypotension or may lose their vital signs altogether. Adherence to ACLS and local protocols coupled with communication with medical control are the key treatment parameters in this extreme event in the prehospital setting.

PNEUMONIA

Pneumonia is the sixth overall cause of death and the leading infectious cause of death in the United States. It is an infection of the lung usually as the result of bacterial, viral, or less commonly, fungal sources and can cause severe respiratory distress in elder patients, particularly those with lung disease or cancer.

The classic patient with pneumonia generally appears ill and may report a recent history of abrupt onset of fever, chills or night sweats, shortness of breath, chest pain, and productive cough or coughing blood. Diagnosis of this condition in elders is difficult, because these findings may not be present. Elders often lack a fever response, and they may not complain of pain or cough. The most frequent findings are increased respiratory rate, decreased blood pressure, and changes in mental status, and none of these are specifically indicative of pneumonia.

The prehospital health care provider should note the duration of symptoms, any change in mental status and medical history. When taking the history, gather pertinent points, such as prior stroke (indicating risk of aspiration), COPD, cancer, diabetes, renal failure, and alcoholism or steroid use. On physical exam, tachycardia, tachypnea, and some degree of respiratory distress may be present. Pulse oximetry may reflect underlying pulmonary disease or a new illness like pneumonia. An abnormal pulse oximetry reading (less than 95 percent on room air) is indicative of a potentially life-threatening condition. Auscultation of the chest may reveal wheezes, rhonchi, tubular breath sounds, or rales. Breath sounds over the involved lobe(s) may be decreased. Right or left upper quadrant abdominal pain may be noted on palpation of patients with infection in lower lung lobes.

Diagnosis and treatment of pneumonia will probably not occur until evaluation in the emergency department is complete. Pneumonia can be diagnosed by x-rays and treated with antibiotics. Most elders require hospitalization for treatment of pneumonia. Prehospital management is aimed at supportive therapy and includes placing patient in position of comfort, administration of supplemental oxygen and nebulized beta agonist as needed for wheezing. An IV lifeline and cardiac monitoring should be established. Patients with respiratory distress or low pulse oximetry readings require high-flow oxygen (10 l/min) by mask. High-flow oxygen therapy should be given to all hypoxic elder patients with suspected pneumonia, even if they have underlying COPD. Many older patients have underlying lung problems such as COPD, congestive heart failure, or cancer that complicate the treatment of pneumonia. Most elder patients are community dwelling and have bronchial or pulmonary infections similar to the younger population. Most cases in the elder population are treated as outpatients without activating the EMS system. Debilitated elder patients are more likely to have recurrent pneumonias. Patients with a history of stroke are at high risk for aspiration pneumonia. The aspiration of foreign material blocks the airways and can lead to pneumonia. Nursing home patients are more likely to become infected with exotic bacteria that have become resistant to routine antibiotics. The prehospital health care provider must be careful to note the presence of and inquire directly about resistant bacteria that has been charted by the nursing home staff. Patients may be carrying bacteria that are resistant to antibiotics: MRSA (methicillin-resistant *Staphylcoccus aureus*) or VRE (vancomycin-resistant *Enterococcus*). These bacteria are easily spread to other patients if simple hand-washing routines are not followed by everyone in contact with infected patients. These bacteria pose no threat to healthy healthcare workers, but if these bacteria cause an infection in an elder person or a person with a weakened immune system, they are very difficult to treat and may cause severe illness or death. Pneumonia is a common source of sepsis or septic shock in elders. Management issues may include establishing IV access to give fluids, or use of vasopressors for blood pressure control and endotracheal intubation in the event of respiratory failure.

PNEUMOTHORAX

Pneumothorax is defined as the presence of free air in the intrapleural space (chest cavity) that collapses the lung on that side. In the atraumatic patient, pneumothorax is classified as either primary or secondary (based on the absence or presence of underlying pulmonary disease, respectively). Both primary and secondary pneumothorax have the potential to develop into a tension pneumothorax, which can become a life-threatening emergency. Because of the specialized nature of this text, only secondary pneumothorax is discussed in this section.

Approximately one third of all spontaneous pneumothoraces are secondary to an underlying pulmonary process and are prominent in the over-40 age group. The most common cause of secondary pneumothorax, implicated in 30–50 percent, is COPD (the combination of emphysema, asthma, or chronic bronchitis). Interestingly, because of the loss of pulmonary elasticity characteristic of COPD, pneumothorax often presents without pain. Dyspnea and anxiety may be out of proportion to degree of collapse because of limited functional reserve. Physical examination is not always helpful, because breath sounds may already be diminished as a result of preexisting lung disease. Less common causes of spontaneous pneumothorax include infection (e.g., pneumonia, tuberculosis, abscess), neoplasm (e.g., lung cancers, lymphomas), and interstitial lung disease (e.g., because of pulmonary fibrosis or autoimmune disease).

Prehospital initial assessment of the elder patient with suspected pneumothorax should include standard ABCs, vital signs, and examination of breath sounds. Focused assessment should include checking for the presence of subcutaneous emphysema, which is a crackling feeling under the skin of the chest or neck caused by air that leaked into the subcutaneous tissues. Establish IV access, cardiac monitoring, and administer oxygen as needed. The presence of tachycardia greater than 140 bpm, worsening hypoxia, jugular venous distention, and tracheal deviation should suggest the development of a tension pneumothorax. This is a true minute-by-minute emergency, and should be treated immediately by needle thoracostomy. This is performed by placement of a large-bore (14- or 16-gauge) needle with a flutter valve in the second intercostal space in the midclavicular line of the affected side. The needle should be advanced over the second rib. The sound of air rushing from the needle indicates the tension pneumothorax has been corrected, and the patient's clinical signs and symptoms should improve dramatically.

HEMOPTYSIS

Hemoptysis (coughing up blood) can cause a great deal of anxiety when experienced by a patient and reflects a range of illnesses from relatively minor to potentially serious. It may not be easy to determine if blood is from a pulmonary source or of nasopharyngeal or GI origin. Blood from the lungs is typically bright red and frothy, with an alkaline pH, whereas blood from the GI tract is often darker, not frothy, with an acid pH and may contain food particles. In rare cases, hemoptysis is life threatening. Hemorrhage in large quantity can impede gas exchange and may ultimately cause death from asphyxiation. Life-threatening hemoptysis may occur when the volume of blood expectorated is greater than 200 cc over a 24-hr period or when pulse oximetry is less than 95 percent on room air. Hemoptysis is usually minor.

Blood in the lungs comes from four potential sources. The most common cause of life-threatening hemorrhage is from bronchial arteries that enlarge in the presence of chronic inflammatory conditions such as tuberculosis, bronchiectasis, abscess, and fungal infections. Rarely, cancerous lesions erode into lower-pressure pulmonary arteries, causing spillage into the lungs. In congestive heart failure, hemorrhage usually stays in the alveoli and is considered serious only when it is severe enough to cause hypoxia. The most common cause of minor hemoptysis is inflamed bronchial capillaries caused by bronchitis or pneumonia. Minor hemoptysis most often occurs when a patient coughs up blood mixed with other lung secretions. Other causes of bleeding into the lung include aortic dissection, PE, or other diseases.

History and physical exam may help in assessing the severity of bleeding but are not always reliable in identifying the cause. The patient's ability to quantify the amount of blood may be unreliable because of their overwhelming anxiety about its presence. Important historical factors include history of lung cancer, tuberculosis, and other previously mentioned diseases and use of medications that may affect blood clotting such as warfarin (Coumadin®) or aspirin. Some patients with massive hemoptysis have unilateral gurgling on exam or have a sensation of warmth in the chest. Vital signs are critical components of the assessment in these patients and can affect management of the problem. Blood pressure is affected only in very massive hemoptysis. In this case, respiratory rate and pulse oximetry become more important. If the patient is unable to clear the airway of blood or is in impending respiratory failure, endotracheal intubation is necessary with a large endotracheal tube (8 Fr or larger). Persistent bleeding despite initial measures is possible, and advancement of the endotracheal tube into the right mainstem bronchus may minimize further aspiration of blood in patients (but only patients with left-sided hemorrhage), but this should be done only under the direction of the medical control physician. Administration of oxygen, establishment of IV access, and cardiac monitoring followed by rapid transport is necessary in the hypoxic, hypotensive patient.

REVIEW QUESTIONS

1. All of the following contribute to the condition of COPD *except*
   a. emphysema
   b. asthma
   c. chronic bronchitis
   d. pneumonia

2. Destruction of lung tissue in emphysema is usually caused by
   a. smoking
   b. pulmonary embolism
   c. pneumonia
   d. inhaled toxins from the work environment

3. Elder patients with COPD can lose their respiratory drive when their blood concentration of _____ is too high
   a. nitrogen
   b. carbon dioxide
   c. solumedrol
   d. oxygen

4. Acceptable prehospital management of suspected COPD exacerbation in the elder patient includes all *except*
   a. breathing into a paper bag to increase blood carbon dioxide concentrations
   b. albuterol
   c. solumedrol
   d. oxygen

5. All are risk factors for a pulmonary embolism in the elder patient *except*
   a. recent surgery
   b. cancer
   c. COPD exacerbation
   d. recent MI

6. Which of the following is suggestive of PE in the elder patient?
   a. Leg swelling
   b. Calf tenderness
   c. High fever
   d. Hemoptysis

7. Elder patients who have had a previous severe stroke are at risk for pneumonia because they may
   a. have resistant strains of bacteria
   b. aspirate stomach contents or food into their lungs
   c. have chronic hypoxia
   d. be bedridden

8. To help reduce the spread of resistant strains of bacteria after handling an elder patient in a nursing home, the prehospital provider should
   a. always wear sterile gloves
   b. always wash his or her hands
   c. take antibiotics
   d. not transfer the patient unless the patient has been given antibiotics by the nursing home staff

9. All are features of a tension pneumothorax *except*
   a. worsening hypoxia
   b. tracheal deviation
   c. jugular venous distension
   d. profound wheezing

10. Proper treatment of a suspected tension pneumothorax is
    a. high flow oxygen
    b. establishment of IV access

    c. placement of a large-bore needle in the midclavicular line, under the second rib on the affected side

    d. placement of a large-bore needle in the midclavicular line, in the second intercostal space, over the second rib on the affected side

11. Hemoptysis in the elder patient

    a. means that the patient must be taking warfarin (Coumadin®)

    b. is always associated with life-threatening illness

    c. can be a symptom of pulmonary or gastrointestinal bleeding

    d. is unlikely to cause anxiety

SUGGESTED READING

Harwood-Nuss, A., ed. 1996. *The Clinical Practice of Emergency Medicine,* 2d edition, Philadelphia: Lippincott–Raven.

Rosen, P. and R. Barkin, eds. 1998. *Emergency Medicine. Concepts and Clinical Practice.* 4th ed. New York: Mosby.

5

Abdominal and Gastrointestinal Emergencies

Mara Stankovich, MD

OBJECTIVES

By the end of this chapter, the prehospital health care provider should be able to:

1 Discuss the importance of abdominal pain as a serious complaint in elders.

2 Identify the factors that predispose elders to gastrointestinal problems.

3 Assess and stabilize the elder patient with an abdominal or gastrointestinal complaint.

4 Develop a working knowledge of the major causes of abdominal pain and their respective complications.

CASE

You are called to the home of an elder woman by her daughter. When you enter her bedroom, you find her lying in bed and her bedclothes are covered with brown, coffee-ground vomitus. She is pale, cool, and slick with diaphoresis. Her daughter states that her mother called her into the bedroom because of stomach pains and vomiting. She states that her mother has had a stroke in the past and takes warfarin (Coumadin®). The mother states that her stomach hurts and she feels weak and dizzy. On examination, her blood pressure is 70 mmHg by palpation and her heart rate is 120. Breath sounds are equal, heart tones are regular but rapid, and the abdomen is distended and feels very stiff, with marked tenderness in the midepigastric area. What do you think is the problem with this woman? What additional questions should you ask her? Is she in danger? What additional treatment can you offer her?

Complaints related to the gastrointestinal tract are among the most common that bring elders to seek medical attention. In evaluating any elder patient, it is important to keep in mind several special considerations that affect assessment and management of this population. They often live alone and without support. They may seek treatment later than their younger counterparts. Abdominal pain in elders is more commonly the result of a serious etiology than in younger patients and more often requires surgical intervention. Mortality from abdominal disease in elders is up to 10 times that seen in younger patients. A complaint of abdominal pain should never be attributed to "an upset stomach" or constipation without thorough assessment. Many elders have other diseases and take multiple medications that may influence the course of the abdominal disease. For example, many cardiac medications may mask the signs of shock. Another example is that elder diabetic patients often have a decreased perception of pain.

The gastrointestinal (GI) tract undergoes changes with age just as the rest of the body does. There is a general loss of smooth muscle tone. Poor tone of the smooth muscle sphincter between the esophagus and stomach leads to heartburn because of acid reflux. Loss of tone along the small and large intestines causes slower movement of intestinal contents and predisposes elders to constipation. This condition may be further influenced by medications the patient may be taking. At the end of the GI tract, the sphincter of the rectum may become weak, resulting in fecal incontinence. The liver, the organ responsible for processing certain drugs and many of the body's metabolic products, shrinks in size. A standard dose of medication may not be sufficiently metabolized by the liver, and dangerous blood levels of the drug may result. Finally, both the inner and outer linings of tract degenerate. The inner lining is involved in the absorption of nutrients. Defects in it may lead to malnutrition. The outer lining serves a protective role. With age, it is less able to wall off inflammation and more prone to perforation. Peritonitis, or inflammation of the abdominal cavity, may develop.

Elders have a decreased ability to sense pain so the *early warning system,* pain before advanced disease, is delayed. Abdominal rigidity, a sign used by medical personnel to detect serious abdominal processes, may not be present because of the loss of abdominal wall musculature. By the time significant pain and tenderness are present, the disease process may be well advanced.

A host of diseases, too numerous for the scope of this chapter, can cause abdominal complaints. This chapter focuses on serious abdominal emergencies commonly seen in elder patients. Nongastrointestinal causes of abdominal pain are mentioned briefly. Assessment of the abdomen is reviewed.

ETIOLOGY

Mesenteric Ischemia

One of the most serious and potentially life-threatening causes of abdominal pain is mesenteric ischemia, which results from an insufficient supply of oxygenated blood to the intestinal tract. Fortunately, it is a cause of abdominal pain in less than 2 percent of cases. It is usually a complication of atherosclerotic disease of the blood vessels supplying the gut, and is primarily seen in the elder population. Medications (e.g., diuretics, cardiac medications) may cause mesenteric ischemia by decreasing flow to the GI tract. Atrial fibrillation and valvular disease of the heart are also risk factors because blood clots resulting from these conditions can travel from the heart and block blood flow in the intestinal arteries.

The onset of symptoms depends on the etiology. Atherosclerosis usually causes a gradual progression of symptoms. There may often be a history of intestinal angina, whereby the patient experiences pain with each meal because more blood is needed during digestion. This demand cannot be met, because blood is unable to flow sufficiently through the partially blocked arteries. If ischemia is the result of an acute event, like a clot suddenly blocking an intestinal artery, the patient complains of the sudden onset of abdominal pain. The patient may give a history of bloody stools, but this is not always a feature of acute mesenteric ischemia.

The hallmark of this disease is a complaint of abdominal pain that is strikingly out of proportion to the findings on abdominal exam. The patient may be in marked distress, but have a benign abdominal exam. Advanced ischemia results in bowel death and cardiovascular collapse. Mesenteric ischemia has a very high mortality rate (85 percent), but this can be decreased if the disease is diagnosed early. Suspect this disease in patients with the risk factors described previously and a relatively normal exam despite complaints of severe pain.

Abdominal Aortic Aneurysm

Another vascular cause of abdominal pain is abdominal aortic aneurysm (AAA). An aneurysm occurs when the muscular wall of the aorta weakens and the pressure from the circulating blood causes an abnormal dilation of the vessel. If this continues over time, there is a risk that the aneurysm will rupture, a catastrophic event that can cause death rapidly from hemorrhage into the abdominal cavity. This disease is more common in elders and in person's with atherosclerosis and hypertension, and males are more commonly affected than females. An intact aneurysm causes no pain. It may be detected as a pulsating abdominal mass on gentle abdominal exam (firm pressure carries risk of causing rupture).

When the aneurysm ruptures, blood leaks out and causes irritation of the surrounding tissues, resulting in pain. Pain is usually felt in the back or in the abdomen and is constant and severe. It may radiate to the pelvis. On examination, the abdomen is firm or even rigid. If the dissection is sufficiently large to decrease flow to the distal vessels, the patient may have decreased or absent femoral and pedal pulses. Rupture of an AAA has a high mortality rate, thus making early diagnosis essential to its successful resolution.

GI Bleeding

Bleeding from the GI tract can be a life-threatening emergency. If the source is the upper GI tract, airway compromise can result. Lower sources of bleeding can bleed briskly and lead to hypovolemic shock. Following is a review of the major causes of GI bleeding.

Peptic ulcer disease. Erosion of the lining of the stomach and duodenum results in ulcer formation and can cause inflammation and pain. However, in the elder population up to 30 percent of ulcers are painless, and the presenting complaint may be bleeding. There is a higher incidence of ulcer disease in the elderly because of their increased use of nonsteroidal antiinflammatory agents (NSAIDs; e.g., ibuprofen, naproxen) to relieve arthritic pain. Use of these agents along with smoking or alcohol are the major risk factors for ulcer formation. If chronic inflammation continues, the ulcer may eventually erode into a blood vessel and cause internal bleeding. The risk of bleeding from an ulcer doubles if the patient is older than 70. Erosion of an ulcer results in vomiting of bright blood (hematemesis) if the bleeding is brisk. Slower bleeding may cause "coffee-ground" hemetemesis and later causes black tarry stool (melena). The blood is partially digested by stomach acids and imparts this color to the vomit or stool. The patient usually complains of sharp epigastric pain and may give a history of similar, although transient, pain after meals. There may be a history of weight loss, as the patient may decrease their food intake for fear of causing pain. Sometimes the ulcer may erode posteriorly and the pain is felt in the back. On physical exam, the abdomen is remarkable for midepigastric tenderness. Vital sign assessment reflects the degree of blood loss.

Esophageal varices. Varices are engorged blood vessels caused by backup of blood flow from the liver circulation. It is primarily a manifestation of liver disease and is seen in patients with a history of alcoholic cirrhosis or hepatitis. Varices are most commonly located is the lower one third of the esophagus. These swollen veins are painless and the abdominal exam is benign. The first sign of presentation is usually massive hematemesis. Signs of accompanying shock may be present if bleeding is rapid. Additional clues to the diagnosis of variceal bleeding are other stigmata of liver disease, such as jaundice or an enlarged liver.

Diverticulosis. Diverticuli are outpouchings or pockets in the wall of the colon and are usually asymptomatic. They are the result of high pressure within the lumen of the colon, usually seen with chronic constipation. They are present in approximately 50 percent of patients older than 60 years because the elastic content of the colon wall changes remarkably with age. Occasionally a diverticulum extends through the path of a blood vessel that is stretched over its surface. The result is painless bleeding and bright red blood with clots in the stools. There can be large amounts of blood lost in the stool with diverticular bleeding. Fortunately, bleeding complicates diverticulosis in only 3 percent to 5 percent of cases.

RETURNING TO THE CASE

Our patient is having a GI bleed. Her rigid and tender abdomen suggests a perforated peptic ulcer. You should ask the family if the patient has had GI bleeding before and whether the doctor had checked her clotting ability recently (because she is taking Coumadin®). You also discover from the daughter that the patient has been taking ibuprofen frequently for arthritis in her knee. She is in shock and has had a lot of bleeding. Recalling the limited cardiovascular reserves of elders, you realize that she is in imminent danger. You place her on supplemental oxygen and place her on the cardiac monitor. You start two large-bore IVs and initiate fluid boluses as you prepare to transport her to the hospital.

Perforation

A perforation or tear in the outer wall of any part of the GI tract can result in leakage of stomach acid, bile, or fecal material into the abdominal cavity. These fluids are extremely irritating to the peritoneum and cause inflammation and pain. Numerous diseases can result in perforation.

Both gastric and duodenal ulcers can perforate through their outer walls, causing sudden onset of excruciating epigastric pain that may radiate to the back. The pain is often constant, and may be accompanied by abdominal rigidity. Inflammation of the intestines can also result in perforation if the inflammation is allowed to progress. For example, in addition to lower GI bleeding, one complication of divertivuli is microperforation of one of the pockets, called *diverticulitis*. Stool leaks out of the defect in the intestinal wall. Patients complain of lower quadrant pain and may also have a fever. Abdominal exam may be remarkable for a fullness or mass in the lower quadrants, most commonly on the left. This is a collection of inflammatory tissue around the contents that leaked out of the colon.

The site of abdominal pain and tenderness depends on where the perforation occurred. The abdominal wall becomes rigid in response to the inflammation caused by perforation, indicating peritonitis. Bowel sounds (assessed by auscultation over a 3–5 min interval) are often absent, because gut motility slows down when peritonitis is present. Nausea and vomiting may occur, and there may be signs of shock if the process is advanced.

Appendicitis

Appendicitis accounts for a relatively high proportion of acute abdominal emergencies in elders. Up to 5 percent of complaints of abdominal pain may be caused by this entity. The presentation and course of disease varies from that in younger patients in several ways. The classic pattern of pain because of inflammation of the appendix is pain first felt in the periumbilical area that later moves to the right lower quadrant. This pattern is present in less than one third of elder patients, who often only complain of vague, poorly defined abdominal pain. Appendicitis has a higher rate of complication in elders. Perforation with gangrene or abscess of the appendix occurs two times more frequently than in younger patients.

Examination of elder patients may not reveal the classic signs of appendicitis. Elders are less likely to have a fever. Abdominal exam may reveal tenderness in the right lower quadrant or diffusely. Vital signs may be normal or indicative of shock if the appendix has perforated and caused sepsis.

Obstruction

There are multiple causes of GI obstruction (blockage of the intestines). One of the most common causes is adhesions, which are the result of prior surgery or intraabdominal inflammation that cause loops of bowel to stick to one another and to the undersurface of the abdominal wall. A tumor inside the intestine can also cause obstruction, located primarily in the large intestine and more common in elders. Tumors may cause slow, lower GI bleeding, or be asymptomatic until large enough to obstruct the passage of stool. Less commonly, a volvulus (twisting of the colon) may cause obstruction. Chronic constipation predisposes elders to stretching and lengthening of the lower part of the colon. This long loop of bowel can twist on itself, resulting in an obstruction. Finally, a large, hard mass of stool can obstruct the lumen of the bowel, resulting in a condition known as *fecal impaction*. This is also more common in elders because multiple factors such as inactivity, medications, and slower gut motility predispose this population to constipation.

An elder patient with obstruction complains of colicky or intermittent abdominal pain. Pain eventually becomes constant if the obstruction has persisted long enough to cause a perforation of the bowel wall. Bowel sounds are variable, depending on the cause of obstruction and the duration of symptoms. Nausea and vomiting of bilious or even feculent material is present because digested material backs up proximal to the obstruction. If the obstruction is lower in the GI tract, significant abdominal distention occurs because air gets trapped between the obstructing lesion and the sphincter of the stomach, which prevents backflow and release of air and pressure. If perforation occurs, the abdomen becomes rigid. Tachycardia and hypotension are often present in elder patients with intestinal obstruction.

Biliary Disease

The liver and gallbladder are the main components of the biliary system. The liver makes bile, a digestive juice, which flows to the intestine to aid in the metabolism of fats. Excess bile is stored in the gallbladder. Bilirubin, a yellow-colored breakdown product of red blood cells, is a major component of bile. Biliary tract disease is the most common diagnosable cause of abdominal pain in elders. Elders are predisposed to disorders of the biliary system for several reasons. Medications may adversely affect the liver, coronary disease may impair blood flow to the area, and the incidence of gallstones increases with age.

Disorders of the biliary system may be manifested by jaundice, a yellow discoloration of the skin and sclera. Obstruction of the normal flow of bile can be caused by gallstones, gallbladder or bile duct tumors, or other obstructing lesions. Patients with liver disease such as cirrhosis are chronically jaundiced, because so much of their liver has been destroyed that they are unable to process bile properly. Painless jaundice can be caused by a pancreatic tumor that blocks the flow of bile into the small intestine. Jaundice may also occur with nonabdominal diseases. For example, congestive heart failure causes blood to back up in the liver, which can lead to leakage of bile and jaundice. Alternatively, increased destruction of red blood cells within the circulation can cause an excess build-up of bilirubin, which stains body tissues yellow. A medical history and list of medications may aid in diagnosing the cause of jaundice.

It has been estimated that 50 percent of patients over 70 have gallstones. In younger patients, common symptoms of gallbladder disease include right upper quadrant abdominal pain after eating fried or fatty foods. In the elder population, these symptoms are not as common. In elders, gallstones are often asymptomatic until they block flow from the gallbladder and cause a build-up of pressure. This blockage results in inflammation and eventual necrosis and inflammation of the gallbladder wall, or cholecystitis. Fever and right upper quadrant pain are the most common complaints. Elders are more prone to the complications of gallstones, which include gangrene, perforation, and ileus (a stopping of gut motility in response to adjacent inflammation). The most serious complication of inflammation of the biliary tract is ascending cholangitis. This occurs when bacteria, usually leaking from the bowel, infect the already inflamed biliary tract. These patients appear more toxic than patients with cholecystitis and often have significant right upper quadrant tenderness and abdominal rigidity. Fever, chills, and vomiting are frequent. The presence of jaundice is required for the diagnosis. Mental status changes or signs of shock may also occur with ascending cholangitis.

Pancreatitis

Inflammation of the pancreas can be caused by many medications or by gallstones that obstruct the flow of digestive enzymes from the pancreas. These enzymes "autodigest" the pancreas and cause significant pain, usually in the epigastric area. Alcohol use is also a risk factor. Nausea and vomiting are accompanying symptoms. Elders are at increased risk for all the complications of pancreatitis, which include hemorrhage, shock because of fluid loss, and infection.

Nonabdominal Etiologies

Besides the diseases listed previously, many diseases outside the abdomen can cause abdominal pain. It is critical for the prehospital health care provider to consider these when evaluating a patient with abdominal complaints. Myocardial infarction (MI), specifically of the inferior surface of the heart, can mimic heartburn or pancreatitis. Myocardial infarction can also present with nausea and vomiting. A cardiac exam and monitoring can aid in differentiation. Upper quadrant or flank pain can sometimes be caused by a lower lobe pneumonia. A history of respiratory complaints such as fever, productive cough, or dyspnea aids in the diagnosis. If in doubt, prehospital personnel should always assume that the elder patient with abdominal complaints may have a serious diagnosis, whether related to the abdomen or another organ system, and provide appropriate monitoring and supportive care.

CASE OUTCOME

When you transfer her to the stretcher, you discover that she has been incontinent of a large quantity of noxious-smelling maroon-colored stool. After 1 l of fluid, her blood pressure increases to 100 mmHg by palpation and her heart rate slows to 105. She becomes less diaphoretic. On arrival at the emergency department, she is further stabilized with a blood transfusion and is taken to the operating room for repair of a perforated bleeding ulcer. She is discharged from the hospital 1 week later and is advised not to take ibuprofen, as this may have worsened her existing ulcer.

ASSESSMENT

Assessing the elder patient with abdominal complaints is often challenging because of dementia, difficulty speaking, and difficulty hearing. This can be further complicated by the fact that many elder patients have extensive medical and surgical histories and may be unable to provide a complete history. When possible, determine any risk factors for serious abdominal diseases. Hypertension and atherosclerosis are risk factors for mesenteric ischemia and AAA. Alcohol use and nonsteroidal antiinflammatory drugs (NSAIDs, such as ibuprofen) are risk factors for ulcers. Time of onset, quality, and location of pain may all aid in diagnosis, but vague complaints are more likely in the elder patient who cannot localize pain as well as a younger patient. Colicky pain is crampy and comes in waves. This is common with obstruction or gallstones. Sudden pain may suggest the rupture of an aneurysm or a perforation. Determine whether there has been any vomiting or any change in bowel habits, including the presence of blood in stools. Although the primary complaint may be related to the abdomen, it is important to do a complete review of systems because of the possibility of a nonabdominal cause of the complaint. Obtain history from caregivers when possible, and always bring medication lists with the patient.

The initial assessment should include the ABCs and vital signs, keeping in mind that a very ill elder patient may have nearly normal vital signs for reasons outlined earlier. There may not be an elevated temperature despite the presence of significant inflammation or infection as the result of the blunted fever response in elders. Tachycardia may not be present in an elder person in the early stages of shock. A normal blood pressure may actually be low for a hypertensive elder patient and may be an indication of early shock.

On focused assessment, make sure to observe the patient briefly before physical examination. In general, patients with peritonitis lie still because even slight movement can increase pain. Patients with colicky pain move around in an attempt to get comfortable. Hydration status can be assessed by examining the mucous membranes. Elders become dehydrated more quickly than others. Assess skin color for jaundice, and look for signs of abuse, such as bruises of varying ages.

Evaluation of the abdomen begins with observation for distention, pulsatile masses, or surgical scars. Auscultation of bowel sounds should be performed. If absent, an obstructive process may be underway. Finally, gentle palpation of all quadrants should be performed to elicit tenderness and assess for peritoneal signs, such as rigidity, as well as for pulsatile masses. Remember that pain out of proportion to the exam may indicate mesenteric ischemia. Assessment of femoral or pedal pulses should be routine.

STABILIZATION AND TREATMENT

The goal of prehospital management of an elder patient with an abdominal emergency should not be a definitive diagnosis. Efforts should focus on attention to ABCs, prevention of complications such as shock or airway compromise, and rapid transport to the hospital, where the diagnostic work-up is best undertaken. Ensure that the patient takes nothing by mouth, including their medications, because this may worsen their condition or cause nausea. Supplemental oxygen by nasal cannula or facemask can be given. A large-bore (18 gauge or larger) intravenous line should be established in nearly all patients to allow for access in the event of shock. This is crucial in patients with GI bleeding who may become hypovolemic quickly. If shock is present or felt to be imminent, two large-bore intravenous lines should be started, although the second one may be started enroute, to minimize on-scene time. Normal saline or lactated Ringer's are ideal fluid choices. Position the patient on their side if they are vomiting to minimize the risk of aspiration. Throughout the entire management of the patient, universal precautions should be maintained.

Ostomies and Feeding Tubes

Many elder patients have had resection of a piece of intestine, most commonly because of cancer or perforation. A surgical opening in the abdominal wall can be created to allow fecal excretion. A bag is placed over this opening to hold the stool. Other patients may require an alternative route to get food into the GI tract if they have difficulty swallowing. A tube can be placed directly into the stomach or small intestine to allow feeding. The outer part of the tube can be seen protruding from the abdominal wall. These are known as *G-tubes* or *J-tubes*. Elder patients who recently had biliary surgery may have temporary surgical tubes in place to drain bile. Some calls to EMS are related to dysfunction of one of these surgical devices. It is best to leave them exactly as they are found and await definitive evaluation at a hospital. Routine supportive care should be initiated.

REVIEW QUESTIONS

1. All of the following are true regarding abdominal pain in elders *except*
   a. elder patients frequently wait longer than younger people before seeking medical help
   b. it is more likely to be the result of a serious or life-threatening problem
   c. it often requires surgery
   d. it is usually not a serious problem

2. All of the following are changes in the GI tract that occur with aging *except*
   a. there is a general loss of smooth muscle tone in the small and large intestine, causing constipation
   b. the risk of perforation is lower than for younger patients
   c. the liver gets smaller and is less able to metabolize many medications
   d. the inner lining of the intestine is less able to absorb nutrients

3. Mesenteric ischemia is a serious cause of abdominal pain in elders that is the result of
   a. diminished arterial flow to the GI tract because of atherosclerotic disease or clot
   b. acute myocardial infarction
   c. bacterial infection
   d. toxic levels of prescription drugs

4. You are called to the home of a 70-year-old man who complains of sudden onset of severe abdominal pain that radiates to the back. He is diaphoretic and has a BP of 60/palpation and HR 130. His abdomen is rigid. You are concerned that he may have
   a. GI bleeding
   b. bowel obstruction

    c. ruptured aortic aneurysm

    d. appendicitis

5. All of the following are common causes of GI bleeding in elders *except*
    a. appendicitis
    b. peptic ulcer disease
    c. esophageal varices
    d. diverticulosis

6. Which of the following can cause abdominal pain in the elder patient?
    a. GI bleeding
    b. Myocardial infarction
    c. Pulmonary embolism
    d. Hepatitis

7. When stabilizing and transferring an elder patient with abdominal pain, the prehospital provider should
    a. establish an IV
    b. provide supplemental oxygen as necessary
    c. allow the patient to drink oral fluids if they are thirsty
    d. place the patient on their side to minimize the risk of aspiration

8. One important way in which elder patients in the early stages of shock as a result of an acute abdominal problem differ from a younger patient is that
    a. elders have a higher respiratory rate
    b. elders always have a temperature
    c. elders may have a normal heart rate
    d. elders have more severe abdominal pain

SUGGESTED READING

Bugliosi, T. F., T. D. Meloy, and L. F. Vukov. 1990. Acute abdominal pain in the elderly. *Annals of Emergency Medicine* 19:1383.

Hunter, G. C. 1989. How to diagnose mesenteric ischemia before it's too late. *Emergency Medicine Reports* 10(20):159.

6

Genitourinary Emergencies

Kyle McClaine, MD

OBJECTIVES

By the end of this chapter, the prehospital health care provider should be able to:

1 Recognize, stabilize, and treat in the prehospital setting elder patients with the following problems:
Urinary tract infection/sepsis
Prostatitis
Epididymitis and orchitis
Fournier's Gangrene
Acute urinary retention
Priapism
Phimosis
Paraphimosis
Complete uterine prolapse
Vaginal bleeding
Hematuria

2 Identify and respond to sexual abuse of elders

CASE

You respond to an assisted-living facility for a man with lower abdominal pain. The nurse tells you that he has been unable to urinate for 12 hr. He is writhing on the bed in pain. He tells you that his urine has been coming out in dribbles all week, and that he was last able to void yesterday. His blood pressure is 190/120 with a heat rate of 110. He is unable to lie still. His abdominal exam shows distension in his lower abdomen. When you press on this area, he states that it worsens the pressure on his bladder. The rest of his abdomen is soft and not tender. What do you think is the problem with this man? What additional questions should you ask him? Is he in danger? What should you avoid doing to this patient? What additional treatment can you offer him?

Elders with genitourinary (GU) complaints frequently use emergency medical services (EMS), both from the home and from other health care facilities. This chapter reviews the causes, evaluation, and prehospital care of elders presenting with GU complaints. The prehospital health care provider should review the evaluation and treatment of elders with shock, a common endpoint for many GU emergencies. Prehospital health care providers should also recognize that GU problems are extremely personal and sensitive issues for elders. Even with a compassionate and sensitive approach on the part of the prehospital provider, elder patients may not be forthcoming about GU problems for reasons of privacy and modesty. Whenever possible, a provider of the same sex as the patient should perform the history and examination. After completing this section, the prehospital health care provider should be comfortable with managing elders requiring prehospital care for GU disorders.

INFECTIONS

Urinary Tract Infections

Genitourinary infections are responsible for 1.6 million emergency department (ED) visits and 100,000 hospitalizations annually. Elders experience more GU infections than both younger adult and pediatric groups combined. The ratio of male to female urinary tract infections changes from approximately 1:30 in the younger adult population to nearly 1:1 in elders because of prostate disease in men. Incomplete bladder emptying and urinary stasis (slowing) arises from compression of the prostatic urethra in the male with an enlarged prostate gland. This results in urinary retention, which interferes with the normal intermittent flushing of the urinary tract. A similar phenomenon exists in older women, with pelvic relaxation, urethrocele, cystocele, and rectocele. These conditions describe the prolapse or herniation of the urethra, bladder, rectum, or uterus from loss of tissue support around the vagina. Urethrocele and cystocele result from relaxation of the anterior vaginal wall, and rectocele from relaxation of the posterior wall. Cystocele and urethrocele, like prostatic enlargement, may prevent complete bladder emptying.

Urinary obstruction may also occur with kidney stones; tumors of the kidney, ureter, bladder, or urethra; and blood clots from urinary tract bleeding. Urinary tract infection (UTI) in elders may also accompany diabetes, the use of immunosuppressive and chemotherapy drugs, use of indwelling devices such as Foley catheters, and exposure to antibiotic-resistant bacteria in hospitals and nursing homes.

When the infection is limited to the urethra or bladder, UTI in elders may present with typical symptoms of urinary frequency, urgency, dysuria (painful urination), and hematuria (blood in the urine), and can be treated in the outpatient setting. More serious infections of the urinary tract can involve the ureter and kidney. Pyelonephritis (kidney infection) with bacteremia (bacteria circulating in the bloodstream) may present in elders without the usual symptoms of fever, chills, and flank pain. Elders may present instead with a change in mental status; gastrointestinal symptoms including nausea, vomiting, diarrhea, and loss of appetite; respiratory distress; or unexplained weakness. The patient may have fever, may have a normal body temperature, or may be hypothermic.

It is imperative for the prehospital health care provider to think of the possibility of early sepsis in these patients. Whenever possible, measure core temperature and check for proper tissue perfusion. Initiate cardiac monitoring and secure IV access in preparation for possible shock. Note tachycardia, tachypnea, or signs of dehydration, which are very significant in the elderly. Treatment en-route is aimed at continual reassessment and management of impending shock.

Prostatitis

In men, the symptoms of frequency, urgency, dysuria, and perineal and low back pain may indicate the presence of prostate infection. This infection often accompanies an acute UTI. Additional symptoms of prostate irritation may include testicular pain, thigh pain, and rectal discomfort. General malaise, fever, chills, arthralgias (joint pains), and myalgias may be present. It is important to note that as with acute UTI, elders with progressive infection or sepsis from prostatitis may present with generalized weakness or with a change in mental status.

Epididymitis and Orchitis

Urinary infections in men may also involve the epididymis and testicle. The epididymis lies in a position posterior to the testicle, and its function is to store immature sperm released from the testicle. Epididymitis occurs most frequently from retrograde travel of urinary bacteria, and may produce impressive symptoms requiring emergency evaluation. The patient may complain of urinary symptoms; lower abdominal, flank, groin, or testicular pain; and scrotal swelling. The patient may have a fever and may appear very ill. On examination, the scrotum may be swollen to twice its normal size, warm and red. This appearance may mimic the presentation of an incarcerated hernia. Other conditions that may give this appearance include tumor, trauma, or early Fournier's gangrene (a rapidly progressive infection of the scrotum).

Evaluation of the patient with possible epididymitis should include an abdominal exam, including bowel sounds on focused assessment. Examination of the scrotum should minimize manipulation. Patient comfort should be maximized and supportive care initiated.

Orchitis, or inflammation of the testicle, is usually associated with epididymitis from direct extension of infection, but may also be caused by other infections such as in mumps in children. In elders, orchitis may be caused by systemic fungal, mycobacterial, or syphilitic infection. Evaluation and treatment are similar to that of epididymitis.

Fournier's Gangrene

Fournier's gangrene is an extremely aggressive skin infection of the scrotum. It is a form of necrotizing fasciitis, an infection that spreads along a defined tissue plane under the skin. Bacteria from an abscess around the urethra or rectum may cause Fournier's gangrene, but many times there is no clear source for this infection. Untreated, it rapidly spreads in the tissue planes under the skin and causes severe systemic infection. The treatment is wide surgical resection accompanied by multiple intravenous antibiotics. The prehospital health care provider should recognize that this is a potentially fatal infection and quickly transport the patient to the ED. As discussed previously, the elder with a serious infection may present with a change in mental status, weakness, or other nonspecific signs and symptoms. Scrotal edema and gangrene with black or blue skin is the hallmark of Fournier's gangrene. Transport the patient rapidly, start IV fluids, and prepare to manage shock with fluid boluses and vasopressors.

EXTERNAL GENITALIA

Complete Uterine Prolapse

For a discussion of the causes and management of uterine prolapse, see the section on vaginal bleeding.

Priapism

Priapism is defined as an acute, painful, and sustained erection not related to sexual desire or stimulation. Apart from the acute painful crisis, untreated priapism results in bladder outlet obstruction and possible impotence because of scarring and destruction of the corpus cavernous (erectile tissue). The most common cause of priapism is penile (intracavernous) injection of papaverine or prostaglandin used to treat impotence. Other causes include malignant tumors of the penis; cancers of the bladder, prostate, testicule, liver, rectum, or kidney; and leukemia. Priapism may result from spinal cord injuries or metastatic cancers of the spine, neurologic disorders, sickle cell anemia, thromboembolic disease, and trauma to the perineum. Priapism has been associated with alcohol use. Several prescription and over-the-counter medications have been associated with priapism, including phenothiazines, antihypertensives, and anticoagulants. Many times there is no identifiable cause of priapism.

Evaluation and treatment of the patient with priapism involves initial and focused assessment and initiation of intravenous access, as the patient may require analgesia and sedation. Acute urinary retention may be present.

Phimosis and Paraphimosis

Phimosis is a narrowing of the penile foreskin that blocks the retraction of the foreskin over the glans penis. Seldom an emergency, phimosis can be congenital and asymptomatic, but may lead to adherence of the foreskin to the glans from fibrosis and scarring and causing urinary obstruction. Irritation can be severe, and may mimic UTI in patients with poor hygiene or chronic urinary catheters (condom or indwelling).

Paraphimosis occurs when the foreskin is contracted and constricted behind the glans penis. This phenomenon is a true emergency, as the constriction causes vascular compromise of the distal penis. Ischemia, necrosis, and gangrene can subsequently occur. Caretakers or health care workers retracting the foreskin during bathing or Foley catheter insertion in elders most frequently cause paraphimosis. Vigorous sexual intercourse or masturbation may cause paraphimosis.

In the prehospital setting, provide pain control and rapid transport to the ED for evaluation and reduction, which may be done manually or surgically.

RETURNING TO THE CASE

This man is clearly suffering from acute urinary retention. This problem is most commonly caused by benign prostatic hypertrophy. The obstruction is usually easily relieved with a Foley catheter. Sometimes the enlarged prostate contains a cancer. The obstructed urine may become infected. Patients obstructed for long periods of time may develop electrolyte abnormalities as well as worsening kidney function. Do not give these patients large boluses of IV fluid; simply monitor the patient and give supplemental oxygen as needed. Urgent transfer to the nearest emergency department is required. A good history is very important, as the enlarged bladder can be mistaken for an abdominal mass or a bowel obstruction.

OBSTRUCTION

Acute Urinary Retention

There are many causes of acute urinary retention in elders, and patients frequently present in great distress. The prehospital health care provider frequently is involved in the evaluation and transport of these patients. Retention may be caused by disease in the penis, urethra, prostate, female pelvis; by drugs; or by neurologic disease. Benign prostatic hypertorphy (BPH) is the most common cause in men. Acute irritation or infection of the prostate may increase obstructing pressure on a urethra that is already constricted by the enlarged prostate. Phimosis with acute inflammation or paraphimosis may cause acute obstruction as well as urethral stricture. In women, prolapse of the urethra because of relaxation or cystocele is frequently the culprit. Fecal impaction may produce enough urethral constriction to cause retention.

Elders frequently take many medications that can contribute to or cause acute retention by central mechanisms. Anticholinergic and adrenergic agonists cause retention by bladder muscle relaxation and bladder outlet contraction, reversing the normal sequence of bladder contraction and outlet relaxation that is required for urination. Medications that cause acute urinary retention frequently encountered by prehospital health care providers include antihistamines and decongestants, such as ephedrine, pseudoephedrine, and phenylpropanolamine; anticholinergic tricyclic class antidepressants, such as imipramine, nortriptyline, and amitryptyline; and amphetamines and phenothiazine antipsychotics, such as chlorpromazine, thioridazine, fluphenazine, and perphenazine. Cogentin, which is used with haloperidol to counteract extrapyramydial symptoms, is also anticholinergic, as are anti-parkinsonian agents, such as bromocriptine.

Neurologic causes for acute urinary retention include spinal cord lesions secondary to trauma or malignancy, cerebrovascular accident, neurogenic bladder secondary to diabetes, or nerve-based infections, such as herpes zoster (shingles). Herpes zoster arises from reactivation of dormant varicella (chickenpox) virus in cranial or thoracic sensory nerve, and often occurs after a viral infection, during stress, or in association with an impaired immune system or chemotherapy.

Symptoms of acute urinary retention may be either obstructive or irritative. Irritative symptoms include dysuria (painful urination), frequency, urgency, and nocturia (need to urinate at night). Obstructive symptoms include hesitancy, straining, decreased size and force or interruption of urinary stream, and sensation of incomplete bladder emptying.

Elders may present atypically. The prehospital health care provider may be faced with an acutely distressed, confused, and agitated patient who cannot localize symptoms. If the patient has been undiagnosed for a significant length of time, he or she may present with acute renal failure from obstruction with additional symptoms from fluid and electrolyte disturbances. The presence of fever and chills may indicate superimposed infection. This is a very important finding, because untreated infection in the setting of obstruction can result in severe kidney damage.

The focused assessment of a patient with known or suspected retention or mental status change should include palpation of the abdomen and suprapubic region for a distended bladder. Provide supportive treatment and transfer to an emergency facility for bladder decompression, management of fluid and electrolyte imbalance, and treatment of underlying condition that may have caused the retention. Analgesia may be required in the field.

CASE OUTCOME

In the emergency department, the patient receives a Foley catheter and 1500 ccs of urine drains rapidly. He is greatly relieved. The bladder distension on physical exam resolves. His kidney function and electrolyes are normal. The Foley catheter is attached to a leg bag and he is discharged back home from the emergency department. He will follow-up with a urologist in 2 days for further care.

GENITOURINARY BLEEDING

Vaginal Bleeding

As women age beyond menopause, changes occur in the external genitalia, vagina, and uterus that lead to frequent complaints requiring medical evaluation. Vaginal bleeding may result from degenerative or pathologic disease in any of these organs.

Elders experience a loss of subcutaneous fat and tissue support throughout the body, including the genitalia. A hypoestrogenic state compounds these changes. Vulvar atrophy and decreased function of Bartholin's glands lead to thinning and dryness of the proximal vagina and external genitalia. Vaginal tissue also thins and atrophies with age, making it susceptible to inflammation and bleeding. Pelvic relaxation, as discussed earlier, can result in herniation of the bladder, rectum, and uterus. The uterus also gets smaller, with the epithelial surface becoming more fragile. The uterus may actually prolapse outside of the vaginal opening and become traumatized, inflamed, and infected. Intrauterine devices, such as pessaries, may erode into vaginal or cervical tissue and cause bleeding. The incidence of uterine malignancy, specifically endometrial cancer, peaks in the elder population, and is by far the most common cancerous cause of postmenopausal bleeding. Cervical cancer may also produce marked vaginal bleeding.

Other causes of vaginal bleeding in elders include: infection of the vagina, cervix, and labia; coagulopathies associated with systemic diseases, such as cirrhosis, hypoparathyroidism, and hypertension; and medications that interfere with coagulation, such as aspirin or warfarin (Coumadin®).

Sexual assault in elders may result in brisk vaginal bleeding. The prehospital health care provider must consider the possibility of sexual abuse in any female patient with vaginal bleeding requiring transport to the hospital. Observations made by prehospital health care providers in the field are a crucial component of complete patient care, and provide clues to guide the subsequent evaluation and disposition of all patients seen in the ED.

The treatment of vaginal bleeding in the elder patient should focus on the management of hypovolemia and shock with intravenous fluid resuscitation. Do not pack anything into the vagina or try to push a bleeding prolapsed uterus back into the vagina. Cover the uterus with a trauma pad moistened with sterile saline.

Hematuria

Hematuria frequently occurs with renal stones or infections of the urinary tract, including urethritis, cystitis, or epididymitis. Renal or urinary stone disease, although less common in the elder population (70 percent of patients with calcium stones present between the ages of 20 and 50), occurs in all age groups. Acute kidney stones may cause typical severe colic-type pain, mental status changes, or distress of unknown origin in the elder patient. Elders may have uric acid stones secondary to gout (25 percent), or calcium stones secondary to hyperparathyroidism, multiple myeloma, or bony metastasis from malignant tumors.

Malignant tumors of the bladder, kidney, ureter, and prostate may produce hematuria. Direct extension of sigmoid colon or rectal lesions into the urinary tract may present with hematuria. A bleeding urethral, bladder, or renal cancer can result in obstruction by bulky clots or the tumor mass itself.

Although usually not life threatening, the appearance of hematuria causes anxiety and concern to patients and caregivers. Malignant bleeding can be significant, and these patients may require resuscitation during transport.

Sexual Abuse of Elders

Elder abuse is a distressing phenomenon that is rarely identified in the prehospital or in-hospital setting. Although this topic is covered in detail in Chapter 17, it is worthwhile to emphasize certain points here. When evaluating and treating elder victims of possible sexual abuse, carry out a careful focused assessment, paying particular attention to the condition in which you find the patient. Note the presence and condition of the patient's clothing. Specifically, look for torn garments and presence of any stains that may contain body fluids. If clothing must be removed for evaluation or treatment of injuries, place them in a plastic bag and keep a document of everyone who comes in contact with them (chain of evidence). If possible, avoid letting the patient drink, urinate, defecate, douche, or bathe to prevent the loss of physical evidence.

Document all visible injuries clearly and legibly. Record in quotation form everything said by the patient during evaluation and transport. Shock, short-term memory loss, self-defensive rationalization, and embarrassment may well interfere with the elder victim's recollection of vital information later. It is imperative that the prehospital health care provider discuss the findings and any physical evidence with the receiving ED physician and nursing staff so that critical documentation and a chain of possession be initiated. If this documentation is not intact or completed properly, the evidence may ultimately be inadmissible in court, further compounding injustice to the victim. The prehospital health care provider has an extremely important role in assuring a positive physical, psychological, and judicial outcome for these elder victims.

REVIEW QUESTIONS

1. Urinary tract infections in the elder population
   a. are less common than in the younger population
   b. can result in sepsis and shock requiring prompt resuscitative efforts by the prehospital provider
   c. are more often encountered in elder men than elder women
   d. usually do not require transfer to the hospital emergency department

2. Urinary tract infections in elders are associated with all of the following conditions *except*
   a. prostate enlargement in men
   b. uterine prolapse in women
   c. diabetes
   d. priapism

3. All of the following are symptoms of severe urinary infection in elders *except*
   a. shortness of breath
   b. change in mental status
   c. vomiting
   d. testicular swelling

4. You are called to the home of an elder man who has had 2 days of pain in the low back and perineal area. He has had difficulty urinating and finally called EMS because he developed a fever and became weak. On initial assessment, his heart rate is 110 and his blood pressure is 140/88. On focused assessment, he has no abdominal tenderness or swelling. You suspect this man is suffering from
   a. prostatitis
   b. acute urinary retention
   c. kidney stone
   d. UTI

5. You are called to a nursing home to transport a man with suspected Fournier's gangrene to the hospital. He is usually alert, but is now confused and has a blood pressure of 90/60. Optimum prehospital management would include
   a. securing his airway
   b. establishment of two large-bore IVs with normal saline or Ringer's lactate
   c. preparing to use vasopressors
   d. all of the above

6. Priapism in the elder male can result from all the following *except*
   a. phenytoin
   b. injection of papaverine
   c. malignant tumors
   d. spinal cord lesions

7. Acute paraphimosis in the elder male may require which of the following from the prehospital provider?
   a. Establishment of two large-bore intravenous lines
   b. Analgesia
   c. Removal of the Foley catheter, if present
   d. Covering the penis with saline-soaked gauze

8. Uterine prolapse in the elder female is a common cause of
   a. abdominal pain
   b. hematuria
   c. urinary retention
   d. vaginal infection

9. Vaginal bleeding in the elder female is associated with all of the following *except*
   a. cancer of the uterus
   b. uterine prolapse
   c. kidney stones
   d. sexual assault

10. Which of the following is true about hematuria in the elder patient?
   a. It is frequently life threatening.
   b. It is associated with UTIs, kidney stones, and tumors.
   c. It usually results in shock.
   d. Is a cause of significant anxiety and concern.

SUGGESTED READING

Harwood-Nuss, A., ed. 1996. *The clinical practice of emergency medicine,* 2d ed. Philadelphia: Lippincott–Raven.

Rosen, P. and R. Barkin, eds. 1998. *Emergency medicine. Concepts and clinical practice.* 4th ed. New York: Mosby.

7

Neurologic Emergencies

John Jardine, MD

OBJECTIVES

By the end of this chapter, the prehospital health care provider should be able to:

1 Define TIA and CVA.

2 Discuss the etiology of cerebrovascular disease.

3 Assess and manage the elder patient with stroke.

4 Discuss the importance of prompt intervention in patients with neurologic symptoms.

5 Define and differentiate the major types of seizures.

6 Assess and manage the elder patient with seizure.

7 Discuss the management of status epilepticus.

8 Define syncope and discuss the common causes of syncope in elders.

9 Define and discuss the possible etiologies of coma.

10 Define AEIOU-TIPS.

11 Assess and manage the unresponsive elder patient.

12 Define confusion and its possible causes.

13 Differentiate the major types of headache.

14 Define and recognize spinal cord compression.

You are called to a nursing home to see an elder woman who was found unconscious in bed by the staff. When you arrive in the room, the patient is unresponsive to voice and pain and is posturing. Her blood pressure is 240/130 with a heart rate of 55 and a respiratory rate of 34. The pupils are pinpoint and nonreactive to light. You start an IV and are in the process of transferring the patient to a stretcher when she has a grand-mal seizure and stops breathing. What do you think is the problem with this patient? Is she in danger? What additional questions should you ask the nursing home staff? Which medications should you consider giving her? Can you offer her any additional treatment? What is her prognosis?

This chapter focuses on changes in the nervous system caused by aging and the neurologic emergencies experienced by elders. Most of the emergencies discussed here become more prevalent with increasing age because of the physiologic effects of aging, a higher incidence of chronic illness in elder patients, their use of a greater number of medications, or a combination of these factors.

The physiologic effects of aging on the central nervous system (CNS) include atrophy (shrinking of brain mass) and decreased nerve conduction time. These changes result in slower reaction times, impaired coordination, impaired balance or gait, and falls. Aging can also affect the senses adversely causing impaired vision and hearing. Elders may also have a diminished perception of pain in comparison to younger persons. As a result of the physiologic affects of aging, elders may also have impaired cognition and short-term memory loss. The degree of CNS impairment varies widely from patient to patient. However, even minimal impairment can become significant or worsen if the elder person becomes acutely ill or injured, or is prescribed certain medications that may have an adverse impact on the CNS.

The neurologic emergencies most common in elder patients are seizure, syncope, stroke, transient ischemic attack (TIA), coma, change in mental status, headache, and spinal cord compression. The clinical presentations, underlying etiologies, and treatments of such neurologic emergencies are often different in elder patients than in other patients and can therefore be more challenging. This chapter discusses pertinent findings of each disease entity. It is assumed that the prehospital health care provider is able to perform a neurologic examination, including AVPU and Glasgow Coma Scales; readers may wish to review this information in a general prehospital care manual. Treatments specific to each of the emergencies are also stressed, but the prehospital health care provider should rely on regional protocols for general guidance.

STROKE

Stroke is the most common neurologic emergency affecting elders and is the third leading cause of death in the United States, after heart disease and cancer. It is the leading cause of disability in adults, affecting nearly 500,000 people each year. Although traditionally considered a physically disabling and frequently lethal disease, recent advances in the acute treatment of stroke are reducing the resultant neurologic deficits and mortality. This section focuses on the definition, causes, clinical presentation and management of stroke.

Stroke, or *cerebrovascular accident* (CVA), is a general term that describes injury or death of brain tissue from the interruption of cerebral blood flow by ischemia or hemorrhage. Ischemic strokes can be further classified as either embolic or thrombotic. Ischemia is caused by reduced blood flow in an arterial blood vessel secondary to an embolus that has come from a larger vessel or the heart, or can be the result of an arterial blood vessel occlusion by blood clot that spontaneously forms at a narrowed or diseased area of a blood vessel (thrombus). An embolus travels from one place to another in the vascular system, whereas a thrombus forms in a particular place and remains stationary. Emboli are usually small blood clots arising from diseased carotid arteries or from the heart. These clots break off and travel downstream until the vessels become too narrow for them to go any further. The embolus then becomes lodged in the blood vessel and prevents the blood from flowing past it. Atrial fibrillation can lead to the formation of clots in the atria that can later embolize to the brain, causing ischemia. Other types of emboli are air, tumor tissue, and fat. Embolic strokes usually occur during waking hours, often without warning. Thrombotic strokes often occur during sleep and are present when the patient awakes in the morning. Most of these patients suffer from widespread atherosclerotic disease, with many areas of blood vessel damage throughout their bodies.

When ischemia occurs in an area of the brain as a result of interrupted cerebral blood flow, that part of the brain stops functioning and the patient suddenly develops neurologic disturbances, such as weakness, sensory loss, or difficulty with speech. If the interruption of cerebral blood flow lasts only a few minutes to 1 hr and is suddenly restored (if the thrombus or embolus is dislodged or breaks up), the part of the brain that had been affected usually resumes functioning and has no permanent damage. This syndrome is called a *transient ischemic attack,* or *TIA.* If ischemia occurs for several hours, the ischemic area of the brain dies and the patient's neurologic disturbances are often permanent. This clinical syndrome is referred to as a *completed stroke.*

A brief stroke-like episode, or TIA, is commonly a warning sign for thrombotic stroke. TIAs temporarily interrupt the blood supply to the brain, producing neurological deficits. To be defined as a TIA rather than a stroke, the deficit must completely resolve within 24 hr. The symptoms of a TIA may last for only a few minutes and may have resolved by the time the patient receives medical attention. Despite finding a "normal" patient on ambulance arrival, the prehospital provider must recognize a TIA as a reliable warning of an impending stroke, and use this window of opportunity to help prevent a major stroke or death.

Hemorrhagic strokes are further classified as either intracerebral or subarachnoid. Onset is usually sudden and marked by a severe headache and stiff neck. Most intracranial hemorrhages occur in hypertensive patients, when a small vessel deep within the brain tissue ruptures. Subarachnoid hemorrhages most often result from congenital blood vessel abnormalities, such as aneurysms and arteriovenous malformations, or from trauma. Bleeding into the brain tissue or subarachnoid space may cause edema and a subsequent rise in intracranial pressure. This may result in further compromise of vital brain functions and ultimately lead to death.

RETURNING TO THE CASE

This patient is exhibiting classic symptoms of an intracranial hemorrhage. Her pinpoint pupils suggest that the hemorrhage is in a part of the brain called the *pons* or the *midbrain*. This is a grave situation. You administer oxygen, establish IV access, begin cardiac monitoring, and give naloxone and thiamine IV. You also check blood glucose, which is normal. There is no change in the patient's condition. While attending to the airway and before intubating the patient, it is important to ask the nursing staff (or family members) if the patient has a living will, advance directive for medical care, or do-not-resuscitate (DNR) order (see Chapter 18). If the patient has specified that she does not want extraordinary measures to be taken, then support the airway with an oral airway and high-flow oxygen, give diazepam (Valium®) IV according to protocol, and transport her to the hospital. If the patient does not have an advance directive or living will, or has specified that she wants "everything done," then intubate her, administer diazepam to control seizures, and transport her to the hospital.

Symptoms of the patient who has experienced a stroke depend on the area of the brain affected by ischemia or, in the case of hemorrhagic stroke, the extent of the hemorrhage. Those areas commonly affected are the motor, speech, and sensory centers. The symptoms of stroke occur suddenly, and the patient may experience seizure activity or loss of consciousness. Respiration may be affected because of paralysis of the soft palate. Speech disturbances may also be the result of paralysis, or may result from direct involvement of the speech center within the brain. Paralysis (hemiplegia) or weakness (hemiparesis) usually involve one side of the body. The patient may also complain of blindness in one eye, difficulty swallowing (dysphagia), gait disturbances, uncoordinated motor movements, or numbness and tingling (paresthesias).

The patient's history is a critical component in establishing the diagnosis of cerebrovascular disease. This is especially true in TIAs, as many patients have a normal examination when the prehospital health care provider evaluates them. Preceding or accompanying symptoms of visual phenomena (lights and sparkles) may suggest migraine. Twitching of the face or extremities suggests seizure. Measuring the blood glucose by test strip or electronic equipment may detect hypoglycemia. A prior history of hypertension, cardiac disease, or sickle cell disease is important. A documented history of a previous CVA is very important, because the deficits found may not be new.

Once stroke or TIA is suspected the prehospital management is primarily supportive. Airway protection must be maintained because paralysis of throat muscles and inability to swallow secretions may compromise respiration. Cerebral oxygenation must be maintained. Suction equipment should be readily available. Administer oxygen with the highest concentration device tolerated; assist ventilation if necessary. If the patient is unresponsive, intubate. An IV should be started, and cardiac rhythm monitored. If hypoglycemia is detected, dextrose 50 percent should be given IV. If IV access is unavailable, give glucagon 1 mg IM. Thiamine and naloxone are reserved for the unresponsive patient. Level of consciousness and degree of neurologic impairment are essential aspects of the neurological evaluation. These may be assessed by the AVPU scale (see the section on unresponsiveness in this chapter for a description) and should be rechecked and documented frequently during transport. Paralyzed extremities should be protected during transport.

On focused assessment, it is important to perform a careful neurologic exam. This should include examination of the pupils, gaze, facial symmetry, speech disturbances, symmetric motor or sensory function, behavior, and orientation. The heart and vascular system must also be thoroughly evaluated, as atrial fibrillation and MI often accompany strokes in elders. Conversely, TIAs are often found in patients with significant coronary artery disease. A search for other injuries is indicated if trauma is historically evident or suspected.

The prehospital health care provider should consider stroke as a critical "brain attack" and bring patients to an emergency facility with the same urgency as heart attack patients. Recent advances in stroke therapy make it even more imperative that patients be brought for definitive treatment quickly. Studies have shown that patients treated with thrombolytic therapy and other neuroprotective drugs within 3 hr of the onset of inschemic stroke may benefit significantly. After 3 hr there is no benefit. Hospitals are developing stroke teams to treat stroke patients rapidly. There are public education campaigns to increase the awareness of stroke symptoms and avoid delaying treatment. Public education, early recognition, rapid prehospital response and new therapies for stroke may begin to decrease the high risk of death and disability associated with this disease.

CASE OUTCOME

The patient has no advance directive for medical care or living will. You intubate her and administer diazepam. The patient stops seizing. A CT scan performed in the emergency department reveals a large pontine hemorrhage. The lesion is felt to be nonoperable. After 2 days the patient shows no improvement, and the patient's family decides to withdraw life support.

SEIZURE

The incidence of seizures increases significantly after age 60, mainly because of an associated rise in the prevalence of stroke, brain tumors, and toxic–metabolic disturbances that precipitate seizures. New-onset seizures in elder patients can pose a significant challenge to prehospital health care providers. Other conditions present similarly at this stage of life. The prehospital health care provider must differentiate seizures from TIAs, syncope, and psychiatric disorders.

A review of definitions may be helpful in assessing elder patients with seizures. A *seizure* is defined as a temporary disorder of the nervous system because of a sudden, excessive, disorderly discharge of brain neurons. Most seizures requiring an EMS call are generalized, involving a loss of consciousness. Most generalized seizures are convulsive, with jerking motions or spasms of the muscles (tonic–clonic activity). Nonconvulsive seizures include brief lapses of consciousness and "drop attacks," which occasionally result in an EMS call. A period of disorientation (postictal period) usually occurs after the seizure. Partial seizures without an alteration in awareness can occur and may evolve into generalized seizures. A patient is diagnosed with epilepsy after the occurrence of recurrent (more than two or three) seizures. An emergency condition requiring careful management is *status epilepticus,* defined as two or more successive seizures without intervening periods of consciousness. If not treated quickly, status epilepticus can cause permanent brain damage.

Assessment of the elder patient with seizure activity involves differentiating events that are true seizures from those that are not. Not all events involving a loss of consciousness, altered mental status, or involuntary movements are seizures. Disorders such as TIAs, syncope, migraine headaches, transient global amnesia, psychiatric and sleep disorders, hypoxia, hypoglycemia, and hypotension may mimic seizures. The prehospital health care provider, serving as the "eyes and ears" of the physician, should carefully observe the elder patient on arrival at the scene. An eyewitness account of abnormal motions or confusion after the event may assist in the definitive diagnosis.

Stroke accounts for 30–50 percent of true seizures in older patients, tumors for 10–15 percent, and other causes for the remainder. Seizures caused by toxic–metabolic disturbances may result from diabetes, renal failure, misuse of sleeping pills or alcohol, or drug interactions. A careful and detailed history from the relatives, witnesses, and/or patient caregivers gives the prehospital health care provider important data that may influence management and diagnosis. Often the prehospital health care provider has more access to relevant data than the emergency physician.

When obtaining a history, the prehospital health care provider should first determine whether there is a history of seizure occurrence. Witnesses should be asked to describe exactly what happened, including the duration of the seizure, whether it was generalized or local, and whether the patient sustained any trauma. Note the presence of incontinence. Record the seizure history, anticonvulsant medications, and recent history of head trauma, fever, headache, or stiff neck. Medical history includes history of diabetes, heart disease, or stroke. When inquiring about the patient's medications, be sure to explore any recent changes in drug prescriptions, as well as any recent alcohol or drug abuse.

The focused assessment of the patient may give clues to the cause of the seizure. Examine the head for evidence of trauma. The neurological exam should occur when the seizure subsides, noting motor or sensory losses. Management of the seizure patient includes attention to the ABCs with airway maintenance and the administration of supplemental oxygen. Most seizures last for minutes and require only supportive intervention. The patient should be positioned on his or her left side after the tonic–clonic phase, with airway suctioning if indicated. Initiate cardiac monitoring and establish IV access. Supportive therapy is all that is required for most seizures; however, recurrent or prolonged seizures create hypoxia of brain tissue and can be life threatening. They require advanced life support interventions as they can result in respiratory arrest, extreme hypertension, increased intracranial pressure, elevations in body temperature, and fractures of the long bones and spine.

The most critical intervention in these patients is airway management with oxygen supplementation. Because air exchange is generally ineffective, ventilation should be assisted with bag–valve mask with 100 percent oxygen. Cardiac monitoring and IV should be initiated. If test strips or electronic equipment are available, determine the patient's blood glucose concentration. If blood glucose is less than 60 mg/dl or unknown, administer thiamine HCl 100 mg IV push or IM, followed by dextrose (D50W) 25 gm (50 ml) IV over 2 min. When IV access cannot be established, administer glucagon 1 mg IM. Give naloxone HCl (Narcan®) 2 mg IV push if narcotic overdose is suspected. If seizures continue, give diazepam (Valium®) 5–10 mg IV over 1–2 min, repeating the dose at 5 to 15 min intervals as needed, with a maximum total dose of 30 mg. Continued seizure activity may require endotracheal intubation and administration of phenytoin (Dilantin®), phenobarbital, lorazepam (Ativan®), or other anticonvulsants according to regional protocols. The use of phenytoin or phenobarbital in the elder patient in the prehospital setting should be done only under direction of the medical control physician. Transport to an emergency facility must not be delayed.

SYNCOPE

Syncope is a sudden and temporary loss of consciousness not caused by trauma or seizures. Elder people are at increased risk for syncope because of the physiologic changes of aging, the higher incidence of chronic illness, and the greater number of medications that they consume, many of which can cause postural hypotension. Although some episodes of syncope are benign and self-limited, patients age 65 and older are at increased risk of injury from syncope-related falls and of sudden cardiac death.

The cause of syncope is frequently difficult to determine. A thorough history and physical examination can reveal the cause of syncope in about half of all patients. Syncope can be classified as cardiovascular, noncardiovascular, or unexplained. Cardiovascular causes can be separated into electrical or mechanical dysfunction. Dysrhythmias such as atrioventricular block, supraventricular or ventricular arrhythmias, long QT syndrome, and sick sinus syndrome represent electrical causes of syncope. Mechanical cardiovascular causes of syncope result from obstruction of central circulation at the level of a cardiac valve or major vascular structure. Several life-threatening entities such as myocardial infarction (MI) aortic dissection, and pulmonary embolus (PE) may also present as syncope.

Orthostatic hypotension is perhaps the most common noncardiovascular cause of syncope in elders. Simply defined, *orthostatic* or *postural hypotension* is a drop in blood pressure with postural change (usually standing from a lying or sitting position) because of hypovolemia or inadequate vasoconstrictor reflexes resulting in venous pooling. Conditions frequently found in elders (e.g., diabetes, chronic alcoholism, diarrhea, gastrointestinal bleeding) can affect intravascular volume. Common medications such as diuretics can cause dehydration, whereas others, such as beta blockers or vasodilators, aggravate age-related inadequacies in vasomotor tone. Nitrates are the most common type of medication implicated in syncope.

Vasovagal episodes are a common cause of syncope in the young but are uncommon in elders. They are caused by a fall in systemic blood pressure from peripheral vasodilatation and slowing of the heart rate. Fright; prolonged standing; hot, crowded rooms; the sight of blood; or defecation can initiate vasovagal syncope. Episodes are commonly preceded by weakness, nausea, or lightheadedness.

Micturition syncope commonly occurs in elder men with enlarged prostate glands. The patient strains during the act of voiding (i.e., Valsalva maneuver), causing a vasovagal syncope. Carotid sinus hypersensitivity can occur with stimulation of special receptors located in the carotid arteries, leading to a slowing of the heart rate and vasovagal syncope. The diagnosis is suspected from the patient's history of syncope during positioning of the head or when wearing tight collars. Neurologic conditions, specifically TIAs, may cause syncope. Seizures may be confused with syncope in elders.

To assess syncope, the prehospital health care provider should obtain a detailed and accurate history of the event by gathering information from the patient and witnesses. Of special importance are accurate descriptions of any preceding symptoms, the patient's activity at the time of the attack, and the course and duration of the attack. The presence of associated symptoms, such as seizure activity, loss of continence, chest pain, dyspnea, diaphoresis, headache, palpitations, or emotional outbursts, should be noted. A general medical history should include similar past events, medications, and drug or alcohol consumption.

Fortunately, the vast majority of patients with syncope rapidly regain normal mental status and have stable vital signs. However, the priorities, as in any medical emergency, are the ABCs. Oxygen therapy and IV access should be initiated. Two large-bore IVs may be necessary in known cases of hypovolemia, such as GI bleeding. Care must be taken not to fluid overload the patient. Cardiac monitoring is essential, as it can provide important information about the patient's cardiac rhythm and the QRS morphology, both of which may help guide further evaluation. Dysrhythmias and ischemic chest pain should be treated with established ACLS protocols.

On focused assessment of the patient, the prehospital health care provider should assess for any trauma secondary to a fall. Elder patients are more likely than others to suffer head trauma during syncope. Carotid pulses should be assessed, with auscultation for bruits. The lungs and heart should be auscultated, with notation of any abnormal sounds (murmurs, rales) suggesting underlying abnormalities. The abdomen should be evaluated for any signs of GI bleeding (the presence of dark, foul-smelling stool, often black or maroon) and gently palpated to check for tenderness. A pulsatile mass in the abdomen is suggestive of an abdominal aortic aneurysm, which can rupture and cause syncope. A careful neurologic examination must be performed, with particular attention to responsiveness, eye movements and pupillary responses, respiratory pattern, motor response and muscle tone, reflexes, and the presence of focal findings. To assess and describe the level of consciousness, the AVPU scale (described in the next section) is preferred in the prehospital setting.

All elder patients who have syncope should be transported to the hospital. Patients with life-threatening emergencies—acute MI, significant dysrhythmias, acute GI bleeding, pulmonary emboli, or drug or medication overdoses—obviously require immediate intervention and may be treated while enroute to the hospital. The remainder of elder patients with syncope also require hospitalization, because the cause, although unclear, is usually serious.

UNRESPONSIVENESS (COMA)

The unresponsive patient may be the most challenging patient encountered in the prehospital setting. Although unresponsiveness is the most dramatic of the disorders of consciousness, it is only an endpoint in the continuum of altered mental status. Any disease process that can cause unresponsiveness may initially present with mild alterations of mental status, which, in time, may progress to unresponsiveness. The prehospital health care provider encounters patients in various stages along this continuum, presenting in a multitude of ways. The mnemonic *AVPU* (alert, verbal, painful, unresponsive) is a simple and useful tool to describe the level of consciousness of an elder patient.

Consciousness is defined as an awareness of self and the environment. Disorders of consciousness can be divided according to levels of patient responsiveness. A patient in a normal state of consciousness is awake and alert. An elder patient who is responsive to verbal stimuli has a depressed mental status in which he or she may appear wakeful but has depressed awareness of self and environment globally and cannot be aroused to full function. A patient who is responsive only to vigorous painful stimuli has a significantly depressed level of consciousness, and appears unresponsive after the painful stimulus has ceased. A patient is unresponsive if he or she cannot be aroused by verbal and physical stimuli to produce any meaningful response. There are only two mechanisms capable of causing disorders of consciousness: structural lesions that encroach on or actually destroy brain tissue, and toxic–metabolic states that alter brain function.

The numerous causes of altered mental status may be divided into the following groups:

Structural	Trauma
	Brain tumor
	Epilepsy
	Intracranial hemorrhage
	Other space-occupying lesions
Metabolic	Anoxia
	Hypoglycemia
	Diabetic ketoacidosis
	Hepatic failure
	Renal failure
	Thiamine deficiency
	Thyroid disease
Drugs	Barbiturates
	Narcotics
	Hallucinogens
	Depressants
	Alcohol
Cardiovascular	Hypertensive encephalopathy
	Shock
	Anaphylaxis
	Dysrhythmias
	Cardiac arrest
	Cerebrovascular Accident (CVA)
Pulmonary	Chronic Obstructive Pulmonary Disease (COPD)
	Inhalation of toxic gas
Infections	Meningitis
	Encephalitis
Environmental	Heat stroke
	Hypothermia

With such an extensive list of possibilities, it may be helpful to use the mnemonic AEIOU–TIPS when evaluating a patient with coma.

A	Alcohol
E	Epilepsy, encephalopathy, environmental
I	Insulin
O	Opiates, overdose
U	Uremia (kidney failure)
T	Trauma, tumor
I	Infection
P	Psychiatric, poison
S	Shock, stroke

The initial assessment of a patient presenting with unresponsiveness should be performed quickly and focus on ABCs and stabilization. The primary concern in any neurologic emergency is always the ABCs with C-spine control. The patient's level of consciousness should be documented with a quantifying scale such as the AVPU scale. The patient's environment should be surveyed for clues about the cause of the problem such as suicide notes, drug bottles, and Medic-Alert tags. If witnesses or caregivers are present, ask them if the patient had seizure activity or had sustained head trauma within the previous year (possibly resulting in a subdural hematoma). When carbon monoxide poisoning is suspected, the prehospital health care provider's safety becomes a concern. The patient should be removed from the hazardous environment after the safety of the rescue crew has been assured.

During treatment of the unresponsive patient, pay special attention to the airway and cervical spine. Unless able to rule out trauma, stabilize the neck and spine with a cervical collar and spineboard while securing the airway. An unresponsive patient always requires an appropriate airway adjunct and supported respirations. Administer high-flow oxygen. Obtain IV access and, if shock is present, begin fluid resuscitation. Monitor cardiac rhythm. If glucose test strips or electronic equipment are available, determine the blood glucose concentration. In patients with blood glucose less than 60 mg/dl or with impaired consciousness of unknown cause, administer Thiamine HCL and dextrose IV. In a patient who is hyperglycemic because of poorly controlled diabetes, the increase in blood glucose concentration produced by the administration of one ampule of dextrose should not do harm. If, however, the patient is hypoglycemic, dextrose is life saving. When IV access cannot be established, administer glucagon 1 mg IM. Reversal of hypoglycemia may fully arouse the patient. Although no further advanced life-support interventions may be necessary, the patient should be transported to a medical facility for full evaluation.

Naloxone should be administered when the patient is suspected of having a narcotic overdose. This may be less likely in the elder population, but substance abuse, especially of prescription medications, does occur in elders. Review the patient's medications and consider naloxone. Specific treatments of unresponsive patients may be dictated by regional protocols.

The history is obtained while stabilizing the patient. Obtain information from bystanders, family, or friends regarding onset of symptoms, preceding events, history of recent head trauma, medical history, current medications, and possible exposure to toxic agents such as alcohol or drugs. The prehospital health care provider has access to witnesses that may not later be available to emergency department personnel. The importance of this aspect of prehospital care cannot be overstated.

The focused assessment of the patient should include a complete neurological evaluation with attention to findings that may be clues to the cause of impaired consciousness. Examination of the patient's eyes may be the single most important assessment in the evaluation of unresponsiveness. Pupils are more likely to remain equal and reactive in toxic–metabolic states; fixed or asymmetric pupils tend to imply structural brain lesions. Dysconjugate gaze at rest usually suggests a structural brainstem injury or alcohol intoxication.

Motor responses to noxious stimuli help detect the level and asymmetry of brain dysfunction. Asymmetry generally implies structural lesions. Appropriate responses, including localization or withdrawal from pain, point to intact cortical functioning. Decorticate and decerebrate posturing are abnormal responses in the unresponsive patient and are ominous signs of deep cerebral hemispheric or severe brainstem injury.

The remainder of the secondary survey should include vital signs looking for relative hypertension and bradycardia. Note odors on the patient's breath, including ketones (indicating diabetic ketoacidosis), or alcohol. Tongue trauma may indicate seizure activity. A general skin exam may reveal needle tracks or jaundice, suggesting liver failure.

The prehospital health care provider must carry out a systematic evaluation while simultaneously stabilizing the patient with altered level of consciousness. Early recognition and correction of reversible causes and other advanced life support interventions may help to save brain function and patients' lives. Prehospital care is completed when a verbal report and thorough documentation of the patient encounter are delivered with the patient. Unless the prehospital health care provider carefully gathers information, significant clues may be left behind at the scene.

CHANGE IN MENTAL STATUS

It is very likely that a prehospital health care provider will receive a request to evaluate an acutely confused elder patient. Clinically defined, *confusion* is the loss of one's capacity to think with usual clarity and coherence. It is a symptom, not a diagnosis, and may be caused by delirium, dementia, or psychiatric disorders. *Delirium* is an acute organic mental syndrome characterized by an attention deficit, rambling or incoherent speech, a fluctuating course, and other manifestations of impaired thinking. *Dementia* is a chronic organic mental syndrome, usually beginning gradually and worsening over a period of weeks to months, and is characterized by memory loss and impaired thinking. The most common type of dementia is Alzheimer's disease, affecting some 2.5 million American adults. An acute episode of delirium may be superimposed on dementia, further complicating the diagnosis.

Delirious patients may be disoriented, experience hallucinations, or exhibit hyperactive behavior and combativeness. However, many elder patients become hypoactive when delirious, with psychomotor slowing, passive behavior, and slowing of speech. These patients may progress quietly to an altered level of consciousness or unresponsiveness.

The most common causes of delirium in elder patients are the use of psychotropic drugs, the presence of a urinary tract infection or other infection, and the presence of underlying dementia in combination with an acute illness. Other possible medical causes of delirium include medications, metabolic imbalances, neurologic disorders (including stroke and seizures), cardiopulmonary disorders, substance abuse, and endocrine disorders.

The assessment of delirium begins with a careful history obtained from family, friends, or caregivers. The patient should undergo a thorough physical examination on secondary assessment, with particular attention to the neurologic exam.

Treatment of the acutely confused elder patient is primarily supportive, after treatable causes such as hypoxia, hypoglycemia, and drug actions and interactions have been ruled out. If test strips or electronic equipment are available, blood glucose concentration may be tested and treated. A calm, supportive attitude may make invasive interventions in the agitated or combative patient unnecessary. Occasionally, the use of restraints during transport may become necessary to ensure patient safety. The prehospital health care provider is encouraged to follow local protocols regarding this practice.

Transport to a medical facility is important, as prompt diagnosis and specific treatment of the acute medical condition are paramount.

HEADACHE

Headache accounts for about 2 percent of all visits to emergency departments. Headaches are less common in elders than among other populations. However, elders may rely on the EMS when afflicted by severe headache.

Severe headaches in elder patients may be a warning sign of a serious illness. Tension headaches tend to respond to aspirin or acetaminophen and seldom prompt an EMS call. In addition, elders seldom suffer from migraine headaches. Nausea and vomiting with headache in an elder patient are ominous symptoms of increased intracranial pressure from hemorrhage or mass. Headaches associated with difficulty talking, tingling of the face or extremities, or actual hemiparesis may be signs of TIA or stroke.

A subarachnoid or intracranial hemorrhage is often associated with the sudden onset of a severe headache frequently described as "the worst headache of my life" and may present with impairment of consciousness or new neurologic deficit. The patient may also develop a stiff neck, nausea, and vomiting in response to meningeal irritation. The headache of the patient with a tumor or increased intracranial pressure is usually slow to develop with a gradual change in intensity and frequency, over many weeks or months.

Temporal arteritis and glaucoma are two other conditions that may present as headache in elders. *Temporal arteritis* is a form of vasculitis causing inflammation of the temporal artery. It commonly presents as headache and facial pain. Untreated, it can lead to blindness. Glaucoma is a disease causing increased intraocular pressure and may present as headache, eye pain, red eye, and vomiting. It, too, may lead to blindness. Early diagnosis of these conditions is critical in preventing blindness.

Always consider carbon monoxide (CO) poisoning in any elder patient complaining of headache, especially in cooler months. One of the first signs of CO poisoning is headache, which may progress to dizziness, vomiting, syncope, seizures, and coma. Ask whether other people who share the elder person's dwelling are also suffering from headaches. Also ask whether the headaches improve if the patient has been outdoors or away from their own dwelling for some time.

In evaluating the patient with headache, a careful history should be obtained, including character and duration of the pain and exacerbating or alleviating factors. As with other neurologic conditions, medical history and medications are also important. Focused assessment of the patient should include a thorough neurologic exam as well as a search for associated signs as described with each headache type. Treatment is supportive, and transport to a medical facility is recommended. Oxygen 100 percent by face mask should be given to all patients supected of having CO poisoning. The prehospital health care provider is encouraged to follow local protocols regarding pain management in these patients.

SPINAL CORD COMPRESSION

Acute spinal cord compression may produce symptoms in an elder patient prompting activation of the EMS and subsequent evaluation by the prehospital health care provider. A patient with spinal cord compression usually presents with a chief complaint of progressive weakness and difficulty walking.

Although spinal cord compression can be caused by a variety of diseases, the most common in the elder population are metastatic tumor, intervertebral disc extrusion, degenerative disease of the bone, spinal stenosis, and trauma. In addition, important diagnostic considerations include infections such as epidural abscess and spinal tuberculosis.

Patients with spinal cord compression may complain of tingling or numbness and weakness in either the upper or lower extremities.

Paresthesias of the upper extremities are most common with cervical cord compression. A change in urinary frequency, as well as constipation and rectal sphincter disturbance, may be described with lower cord compression. Bowel and bladder incontinence are poor prognostic signs that may indicate advanced and irreversible compression. Gait disturbances and falling are common and are associated with motor weakness of the lower extremities. Many patients also have focal pain at the site of compression in the spine.

Focused assessment of these patients should include a thorough neurologic exam. During the physical exam, any evidence of trauma should be noted. Treatment is supportive, but transport to a medical facility is imperative. Spinal cord compression is a neurologic emergency that can result in irreparable damage if not treated aggressively. All patients should be carefully C-spine immobilized prior to hospital transfer. Intravenous steroids are used to decrease inflammation and edema in the area of compression. The prehospital health care provider should consult local protocols and medical control for this treatment option. Definitive therapy may require surgery, radiation therapy, or both.

REVIEW QUESTIONS

1. The most common acute neurologic emergency in elder Americans is
   a. TIA
   b. stroke
   c. seizure
   d. change in mental status

2. An ischemic stroke can result from interruption of cerebral blood flow from all of the following *except*
   a. blood clot
   b. air emboli
   c. fat emboli
   d. hemorrhage

3. All of the following are true about a TIA *except*
   a. It can be considered a warning sign for a future stroke.
   b. The symptoms will completely resolve in 24 hr or less.
   c. It is usually hemorrhagic in elders.
   d. All patients with suspected TIA should be transported to the closest emergency facility.

4. Which of the following are often associated with stroke in elders? (Choose all that apply.)
   a. Hypoglycemia
   b. Atrial fibrillation
   c. Coumadin use
   d. Recent MI

5. Elder patients with a suspected stroke or "brain attack" may be eligible to receive thrombolytic therapy or other neuroprotective drugs. To benefit from these medicines, these patients should be transported to the emergency department within _____ hr(s) of the beginning of their symptoms
   a. 1
   b. 3
   c. 6
   d. 8

6. All of the following can contribute to the increased seizure risk in the elder population *except*
   a. stroke
   b. tumors
   c. toxic–metabolic disturbances
   d. diabetes

7. Most seizures in elders require
   a. diazepam 5–10 mg IV
   b. supportive care
   c. phenobarbital 30 mg IV
   d. dextrose (D50W) 25 gm IV

8. Syncope resulting from orthostatic or postural hypotension in the elder population is usually the result of
   a. multiple medications
   b. ventricular arrhythmias
   c. TIA/CVA
   d. dehydration

9. It is critical for the prehospital provider to remember which of the following when assessing an elder patient with unresponsiveness?
   a. They have usually had a hemorrhagic stroke.
   b. They can be given oral glucose preparations safely.
   c. Glucagon 1.0 mg should be given to all unresponsive patients.
   d. Information obtained from family and bystanders is critical to discovering the cause of unresponsiveness.

10. All of the following are causes of headache commonly seen in the elderly *except*
    a. temporal arteritis
    b. glaucoma
    c. intracranial hemorrhage
    d. migraine headache

SUGGESTED READING

Harwood-Nuss, A., ed. 1996. *The clinical practice of emergency medicine.* 2d ed. Philadelphia: Lippincott–Raven.

Endocrine Emergencies

Masood Khan, MD, and John E. Morley, MB, BCh

OBJECTIVES

By the end of this chapter, the prehospital health care provider should be able to:

1 Describe common endocrine emergencies in the elder population.
2 Describe basic pathophysiology and clinical manifestations of endocrine emergencies affecting elders.
3 Identify risk factors for endocrine emergencies in the elder patient.
4 Assess and stabilize the elder patient with a suspected endocrine emergency.

You are called to the scene of a minor car accident. When you arrive, you find a man crouched behind the wheel of a large automobile. He has run into a telephone pole, but there is only minor damage to the front bumper. The patient is wearing a seatbelt and muttering incoherently. He does not acknowledge you when you approach the car. He is drenched in a cold sweat that soaks his clothing. His grandson, a teenager, is with him in the car and is uninjured. The grandson states that the patient seemed fine when they began driving, but then became increasingly confused. What do you think is the problem with this man? Is he in danger? What additional questions should you ask his grandson? What treatment can you offer him? Are there any medications you should consider giving him? If so, what are the appropriate dosages?

Nutritional and endocrine disorders occur commonly in elder persons and may present as acute emergencies. Endocrine disorders that present with a sudden change in mental status frequently result in activation of the emergency medical system (EMS). The prehospital health care provider should be prepared to identify and manage acute endocrine emergencies in elders. Table 8.1 lists the common endocrine disorders that the prehospital health care provider should consider when evaluating the elder patient with acute confusion (delirium).

DIABETES MELLITUS

Diabetes mellitus (DM) is a clinical syndrome characterized by high serum blood sugars (hyperglycemia) as a result of a deficiency of insulin production by the islets of Langerhans in the pancreas, a

Table 8.1. Endocrinologic Causes of Acute Confusion (Delirium)

Diabetic coma
   Hyperglycemic coma
      Hyperosmolar coma
      Diabetic ketoacidosis (DKA)
      Lactic acidosis
   Hypoglycemic coma
Hypothyroidism
Hyperthyroidism
Addison's disease (hypoadrenalism)

reduction in its biologic effectiveness (insulin resistance), or both. DM has an estimated prevalence of 18 percent in persons older than 65 years in the United States, making DM the most common endocrine problem afflicting the elder population. Elder diabetics may activate the EMS system because they have an emergency that is caused directly by their DM (e.g., hyperglycemia, hypoglycemia), or because they have an emergency that may result from underlying DM (e.g., heart disease, infections).

The human and economic impact of diabetes is staggering. Because DM can affect almost any organ system over time, elders are at particular risk for many of the long-term complications of this disease. Twenty-five percent of all new cases of end-stage renal disease and more than half of all lower extremity amputations occur as a complication of DM. Diabetics have an increased risk of coronary disease, and approximately half of all type II diabetics die as a result of coronary disease. Diabetes is also a leading cause of blindness, with approximately 5,000 new cases per year. DM can also cause chronic painful peripheral neuropathies or sensory loss, especially of the lower extremities. This puts patients at risk for inadvertent injury and infection. Diabetic patients account for 10 percent of all acute care hospital days.

Diabetes is seen worldwide, and the incidence of primary diabetes is rising. Primary diabetes is further categorized into insulin dependent diabetes mellitus (IDDM), or type 1 diabetes, and non-insulin dependent diabetes (NIDDM), or type 2 diabetes. Type 2 diabetes is also known as adult-onset diabetes and is more common in the elder population than type 1. Table 8.2 illustrates characteristics of type 1 and type 2 diabetes.

Table 8.2. Comparison of Type 1 and Type 2 Diabetes

Type 1 (IDDM)	Type 2 (NIDDM)
Usually occurs under 30 years of age	Less than 40 years of age, late and maturity onset obese (50–90 percent)
Early and juvenile onset—nonobese, but 10 percent of persons over 68 years with diabetes have elevated serum ketones and acidosis	No serum ketones or acidosis
Severe endogenous insulin deficiency	Moderate endogenous insulin deficiency Have insulin resistance
Treatment with insulin always necessary	Treatments other than insulin (diet, oral agents) often effective
Associated with other autoimmune diseases	Not associated with other autoimmune diseases

IDDM, Insulin dependent diabetes mellitus; NIDDM, non-insulin dependent diabetes mellitus.

CRITERIA FOR THE DIAGNOSIS OF DIABETES

The prehospital health care provider should be familiar with the symptoms associated with DM and the criteria that physicians use to make the diagnosis of DM. Any one of the following is considered diagnostic of DM:

1. Presence of classic symptoms of diabetes, such as polyuria (increased urine output), polydipsia (increased thirst), ketonuria (presence of ketones in the urine), and rapid weight loss, together with a random glucose elevation (elevation of plasma glucose greater than 200 mg/dl).

2. Elevated fasting glucose concentrations on more than one occasion, venous plasma glucose greater than 126 mg/dl (previously, the fasting value was 140 mg/dl).

3. Fasting glucose concentrations less than that which is diagnostic of diabetes (i.e., 126 mg/dl), but a sustained elevation of glucose concentration during oral glucose tolerance test on more than one occasion (venous plasma glucose of >200 mg/dl).

Diabetes Mellitus—Pathophysiology

Hyperglycemia in elder diabetic patients develops because of absolute insulin deficiency (IDDM) or relative insulin deficiency (NIDDM). Both of these conditions cause reduced rate of removal of glucose from the blood by body tissues and an increased rate of release of glucose from the liver into the circulation. As blood glucose rises, elder patients develop numerous symptoms. Table 8.3 lists the symptoms of acute hyperglycemia in elders.

Many of the symptoms of diabetes are the result of urinary losses of glucose. In the normal patient, glucose is not lost in the urine. In the diabetic patient, when plasma glucose concentrations exceed the ability of the kidneys to reabsorb glucose, then glucose (along with free water and electrolytes) is lost in the urine. The high concentration of glucose in the urine pulls extra free water from the bloodstream into the urine, causing both increased urination (polyuria) and increased loss of free water from the body. Thirst (polydipsia) is a consequence

Table 8.3. Acute Symptoms of Hyperglycemia

Fatigue	Polyuria (increased urination)
Weight loss	Polyphagia (increased appetite)
Blurred vision	Polydipsia (increased thirst)

of losing fluids and electrolytes. Blurred vision develops as the lenses and retinas are exposed to high circulating glucose levels.

Each gram of urinary glucose represents approximately 4.5 Kcal. A poorly controlled elder diabetic spilling 100 g of glucose per day in the urine loses 450 Kcal/day. This amount is enough to cause weight loss and stimulation of food intake (polyphagia). Decreased plasma volume produces dizziness and weakness because of postural hypotension. Hypotension (shock) in the recumbent position is a serious sign. Loss of subcutaneous fat and muscle wasting with fatigue are features of more slowly developing insulin deficiency. When insulin deficiency is absolute and sudden in onset, the symptoms discussed here can progress rapidly.

Insulin is required to transport glucose across cell membranes to be used as fuel by the cell. When insulin deficiency is severe, as is seen in type 1 and some type 2 diabetics, cells are unable to use glucose as fuel, so the liver reacts by breaking down fats into ketones for the cells to use as energy. This causes *ketoacidosis* (accumulation of ketones and acid in the bloodstream), which worsens dehydration by producing *anorexia* (decreased desire to eat), nausea, and vomiting.

Many patients with type 2 diabetes present initially with increased urination and thirst, although others are relatively asymptomatic. This is particularly true in obese patients. Chronic skin infections, especially of the lower extremities, are common in this population. Elder patients who have had a history of frequent lower extremity infections or wounds that are slow to heal may later be diagnosed with type 2 diabetes.

Management of diabetes mellitus may require only a weight-reducing, heart-healthy diet. In many patients, oral drugs may be sufficient to control type 2 diabetes mellitus. Table 8.4 lists commonly prescribed oral hypoglycemics. The prehospital health care provider should be able to readily identify commonly prescribed oral hypogycemic agents to care properly for the elder patient. Insulin

Table 8.4. Oral Agents Available for Treatment of Diabetes Mellitus

Drugs increasing insulin secretion
  Sulfonylureas
    Glyburide (Diabeta®, Glynase®, Micronase®)
    Glipizide (Glucotrol®)
    Glimepride (Amaryl®)
  Nonsulfonylureas
    Repaglinide (Prandin®)
Drugs modulating glucose absorption
  Alpha-1-gluconidase inhibitors, e.g. acarbose (Precose®)
Drugs decreasing insulin resistance
  Biguanides [e.g., metformin (Glucophage®)]

injections are required for all type 1 diabetics and many type 2 diabetics. Insulin may be short-acting (regular) or long-acting (lente, semi-lente, NPH). Mixtures of short-acting and long-acting insulin are available. Most elder patients require two injections of insulin each day.

DIABETIC COMA

Coma in the elder patient with diabetes mellitus can result when blood sugar is too high or too low or as a complication of diabetic infections or shock. *Hyperglycemic coma* is caused by either severe insulin deficiency (resulting in diabetic ketoacidosis) or mild to moderate insulin deficiency (resulting in hyperosmolar hyperglycemic non-ketotic coma). *Hypoglycemic coma* (insulin shock) results from an excessive dose of insulin or hypoglycemic agents. This condition frequently results if a diabetic patient does not eat properly after administering insulin or an oral hypogycemic. *Lactic acidosis* can cause coma in elder diabetics in association with severe infections or with cardiovascular collapse.

DIABETIC KETOACIDOSIS

Diabetic ketoacidosis (DKA) is usually a complication of type 1 diabetes, and therefore is usually seen in younger people. However, elder patients may develop diabetic ketoacidosis. Ten percent of persons more than 60 years of age which are newly diagnosed with diabetes are type 1 diabetics, and the first time this comes to medical attention may be because they have developed DKA. Thus, EMS providers may encounter an elder patient with DKA as their presenting condition, even if that patient was not previously known to be a diabetic.

Diabetic ketoacidosis may also occur in an elder patient who is known to be a type 1 diabetic. Elder patients with type 1 diabetes may suddenly require larger doses of insulin to control their blood glucose. If they do not monitor their own blood glucoses, they may be unaware of this increased insulin requirement, and develop DKA as a result of being insulin deficient. DKA is commonly triggered in type 1 diabetics by myocardial infarction, stroke, infection, loss of appetite, or by stopping or drastically reducing the usual insulin dosage. Poor compliance with insulin is the most common cause of DKA, particularly when episodes are recurrent. Elder persons with DKA have a very high mortality rate. DKA has also been found to be a serious complication of insulin pump therapy, possibly because of pump failure or insulin leakage. In addition, elderly type 2 diabetics may develop DKA as a result of severe infection, which can produce severe insulin deficiency.

Diabetic ketoacidotic coma is characterized by glucose greater than 250 mg/dl, acidosis (blood pH <7.2) and elevated plasma ketone concentration. Hyperglycemia is secondary to insulin deficiency, and leads to both an increase in glucose production by the liver and a decrease in peripheral glucose utilization by the cells. Plasma ketone levels rise because of overproduction by the liver. The classic fruity smell of ketones may be noted on the breath of the comatose diabetic patient.

Assessment

Patients with DKA usually present after several days of polyuria and polydipsia (remember that hyperglycemia produces an osmotic diuresis that results in volume depletion and urinary loss of electrolytes) associated with marked fatigue, nausea, vomiting, anorexia, and occasionally abdominal pain. The abdominal pain sometimes may mimic an acute abdomen. Abdominal tenderness may be present even in the absence of abdominal disease.

On initial assessment, patients may be tachypneic. On focused assessment, patients with DKA typically exhibit dehydration, fruity breath odor of acetone (acetone halitosis), and an altered mental status ranging from disorientation to coma. Kussmaul's respirations (deep sighing respirations) are usually present when the acidosis is severe. Hypotension with tachycardia indicates a critically ill elder patient with profound fluid and electrolyte depletion. Mild hypothermia is usually present.

LABORATORY AND CLINICAL DIAGNOSIS

Clinical diagnosis in the hospital setting is confirmed by demonstration of elevated blood glucose levels, ketones in the blood or urine, glycosuria (presence of glucose in the urine), low blood pH, and low plasma bicarbonate. In the prehospital setting, the fingerstick glucose is high (>250 mg/dl), and clinical features described previously are present.

Stabilization and Treatment

Stabilization of the elder diabetic patient in the field is a key component of treatment. Intravenous fluids (normal saline) should be started, a glucose level checked, and oxygen administered. Always consider the possibility of a fall or trauma prior to the onset of coma, and place the patient in C-spine immobilization if indicated. The patient should be placed on a cardiac monitor. Patients with DKA may have very high serum levels of potassium as a result of accumulation of acid in the blood, and may develop life-threatening cardiac arrhythmias, including ventricular tachycardia or ventricular fibrillation. As a result of the aging process, an elder person's heart may be less able to tolerate the accumulation of acid in the blood that occurs in DKA, and the heart may pump less effectively, which worsens hypotension. Despite the accumulation of acid in the bloodstream in DKA, treatment of DKA with bicarbonate is not indicated in the prehospital setting, neither for elders nor for younger people. The use of bicarbonate in the management of DKA is done only in the hospital setting and only rarely, when the acidosis is particularly severe. Monitor the cardiac rhythm and vital signs closely, and transport the patient to the closest emergency department immediately. Once in the hospital, if the acidosis and ketosis is severe, the patient is admitted to the intensive care unit after emergency evaluation and stabilization. During transport, clinical status and vital signs must be assessed frequently and carefully. The patient should not receive sedatives or narcotics.

Patients with DKA are always dehydrated and hypovolemic. IV fluids are critical in the early treatment of DKA. The average fluid deficit in an adult is 6 l. Rapid volume expansion is usually required. This is best begun by administration of normal saline at a rate of 1 l/hr. In the prehospital setting, 1 l of normal saline would be the maximum that should be administered to the elder patient in DKA, unless transport time is unusually long. For elder patients with renal and cardiovascular disease, slower rates of administration may be necessary to avoid causing sudden pulmonary edema. In the emergency department, after the delivery of 2 l of normal saline, if there are no signs of orthostatic hypotension, the rate of fluid administration can be decreased, and the solution switched to half-normal saline.

Education of diabetic patients to recognize the early symptoms and signs of ketoacidosis has done a great deal to prevent severe acidosis. Patients may check their urine with testing strips for the presence of urinary ketones (ketonuria), especially when the patient has signs of infection or when blood glucose is unexpectedly and persistently high. The patient should be instructed to contact his or her physician or to activate the EMS system if hyperglycemia or ketonuria persists and especially if vomiting develops. If the patient has detected urinary ketones, this information may be reported to the medical control physician.

HYPEROSMOLAR HYPERGLYCEMIC COMA

Hyperosmolar hyperglycemic coma is more common in the elderly diabetic population than the younger population. Prehospital providers are more likely to encounter elder diabetic patients with hyperosmolar hyperglycemic coma than with DKA because hyperosmolar hyperglycemic coma is usually associated with adult-onset (type 2) diabetes. This condition occurs as a result of moderate insulin deficiency, rather than total lack of insulin, as well as decreased responsiveness to circulating insulin in the bloodstream. The onset of symptoms in this illness is slower than in DKA. Elder patients with hyperosmolar hyperglycemic coma have very high blood glucoses and profound dehydration. These patients classically present with a history of polydipsia, followed by dizziness, confusion, and later, coma. Serum blood glucose levels can reach 1000–2000 mg/dl. Prehospital treatment of hyperosmolar hyperglycemic coma involves protecting the airway, establishing one or two large-bore IV lines with normal saline, administering supplemental oxygen, and carefully monitoring cardiac rhythm and vital signs. Despite profound dehydration, extreme care must be taken not to replace fluids too rapidly in elder patients with hyperosmolar hyperglycemic coma because of underlying cardiac disease and the risk of congestive heart failure if IV fluid is given too rapidly. In addition, overly aggressive IV fluid resuscitation can cause serum sodium levels to change too quickly and result in seizures in the elder patient.

RETURNING TO THE CASE

This patient is exhibiting a change in mental status. In the setting of trauma, you must consider head injury. You secure the patient's airway and place him on a cardiac monitor. You then attempt to extricate the patient and place him on a backboard with a rigid cervical collar. He becomes agitated and hostile. During this process, the grandson tells you that his grandfather is diabetic and skipped his usual midday meal because they were out fishing. You are concerned that the patient may be having a hypoglycemic reaction. You give the patient an oral glucose preparation and, with some difficulty, start an IV, draw one tube of blood, and check a fingerstick glucose. His fingerstick glucose is low, and you push 25 cc of D50W. The patient's mental status quickly improves, and he agrees to be transported to the hospital with full C-spine immobilization. No traumatic injuries are identified on focused assessment.

HYPOGLYCEMIC COMA

Hypoglycemic coma occurs when an elder patient receives too much insulin or if an oral hypoglycemic agent has been taken without adequate food intake. Persons are rarely symptomatic before the blood glucose falls below 40 mg/dl; unconsciousness can occur below 30 mg/dl. Confusion and subsequently coma occur because brain cells are deprived of glucose. Most of the early signs of a falling glucose level are the result of activation of the sympathetic nervous system, and include tachycardia, palpitations, excessive sweating, and dizziness. In elder persons, these symptoms may be blunted because of impaired autonomic response associated with age. When hypoglycemia occurs while a person is sleeping, he or she may remember having severe nightmares.

Hypoglycemia in the elder patient is a true emergency. When hypoglycemia is suspected, treatment must be instituted instantly. A blood glucose level should be checked by the fingerstick technique using a glucometer when available. If the person is awake, they should be given orange juice or candy. If the patient is unresponsive, confused, cannot take fluid by mouth, or has no gag reflex, the treatment of choice is 25 cc of 50 percent glucose intravenously. If IV access cannot be obtained, then 1 mg of glucagon IM may be given. Once IV access is established and the patient is responsive, he or she can be given 5 percent glucose intravenously at a rate of approximately 75–100 cc per hr. This is done to prevent recurrence of the hypoglycemic episode.

CASE OUTCOME

The blood glucose from the tube of blood you obtained when you started the IV was 35 mg/dl. You find out from the grandson that he is taking an oral hypoglycemic agent for his diabetes. These agents are very long lasting, so after his workup was completed, he was admitted to the hospital overnight for monitoring of his blood sugar. He was discharged the next day.

OTHER ENDOCRINE DISORDERS

Thyrotoxicosis (Hyperthyroidism)

Thyrotoxicosis is a clinical condition caused by excess secretion of thyroid hormone. It can result from a number of different disorders. The exact incidence of hyperthyroidism in elders is not known, but it is much lower than the incidence of hypothyroidism. Graves disease is an autoimmune disorder resulting in enlargement of the thyroid gland and overproduction of thyroid hormone. Graves disease is the most common cause of hyperthyroidism in elders. Other causes are single or multinodular goiter (enlarged thyroid). Iodine-induced hyperthyroidism (contrast study) and iodine-containing drugs (e.g., amiodarone) can cause both hypothyroidism and hyperthyroidism.

The clinical presentation of the elder thyrotoxic patient is extremely variable. Clinical features depend on the age at onset, duration of illness, and the degree of hormone excess. Symptoms such as heat intolerance, diarrhea, weight loss, and restlessness, which are commonly seen in the younger age group, are seen less commonly in elders. At least 30 percent complain of anorexia and, less commonly, constipation. Prolonged disease is associated with features of chronic catabolism (breakdown of proteins). Skeletal muscle wasting, especially of the limb girdles, induces a proximal muscle weakness. A patient may experience difficulty in climbing stairs or getting up from a sitting position. Thyrotoxic patients commonly experience dyspnea, and although this is usually in the absence of cardiac failure, more severe disease can be manifested by a severe cardiomyopathy and congestive heart failure. This is especially true in elders. One-third of patients present with atrial fibrillation. Elder patients with preexisting angina often complain of worsening angina pectoris.

The mental and emotional changes seen in thyrotoxicosis include anxiety, irritability, poor concentration, restlessness, and emotional lability. In addition, insomnia and forgetfulness are also common in elder patients with hyperthyroidism. Elder patients with thyrotoxicosis are often difficult to diagnose clinically. Focused assessment may reveal a large goiter (enlarged thyroid gland) at the base of the neck anteriorly, although this is not always present in thyrotoxicosis. Tachycardia is also frequently present. Although thyrotoxicosis may be suspected, it is not possible to make this diagnosis definitively in the prehospital setting. Prehospital management includes IV access, careful cardiac monitoring, attention to vital signs, checking a rapid glucose determination, and treatment of unstable cardiac rhythms or congestive heart failure, if present.

HYPOTHYROIDISM

Hypothyroidism is primarily a disease of those age 50 and older, and is more common in women. Spontaneous hypothyroidism in the elderly is sometimes due to thyroiditis that occurs earlier in life and is associated with progressive destruction of gland tissue.

The symptoms and signs of hypothyroidism are often overlooked because complaints such as fatigue, memory loss, and decreased hearing are ascribed to aging without further investigation. The most common symptoms of hypothyroidism include cold intolerance, constipation, dry skin, and lassitude. Other features include fatigue, weight gain, poor concentration, and muscle and joint pains. The skin is dry and scaly, and hair loss is frequent. The voice becomes hoarse and rough. Elder hypothyroid patients often exhibit mental status changes, confusion, paranoia, depression, and dementia. These complaints are also frequently misattributed to the aging process. Nerve entrapment syndromes are also common. Examples include deafness and hand paresthesias (median nerve distribution) because of carpal tunnel syndrome.

On focused assessment, the elder patient with hypothyroidism may have bradycardia; dry, coarse skin; husky voice; loss of eyebrows;

and a non-pitting edema as well as facial edema. Coexisting diseases, such as congestive heart failure, may present with pitting edema.

Prehospital management of hypothyroidism is similar to that of hyperthyroidism. In-hospital treatment of hypothyroidism includes stepwise replacement of thyroid hormone. Treatment should be started at 0.050 mg sodium levothyroxine (Synthroid®) per day and the dose increased by 0.025 mg at 2 to 4-week intervals to a maintenance dose of 0.75–0.1 mg. The physician monitors heart rate response and symptoms of angina. In elder persons with heart disease or chronic obstructive pulmonary disease, slightly lower doses may be associated with symptomatic improvement.

Myxedema coma is a fatal complication of hypothyroidism in elder persons. The clinical picture includes hypothermia, altered mental status, and coma. Precipitating events include surgery, hypothermia, infection, hypoglycemia, and sedative drugs. A scar on the neck from previous surgery is a clue to the cause of coma. Because the patient with this disorder can die of respiratory failure (CO_2 narcosis), prompt attention to airway stabilization and management in the prehospital setting is paramount. Again, although this diagnosis may be suspected in the elder comatose patient, it cannot be confirmed until the patient is in the in-hospital setting. These patients should be managed like any other unresponsive patient in the prehospital setting with airway control, endotracheal intubation, cardiac monitoring, careful assessment and monitoring of vital signs, IV fluid administration, and assessment of blood glucose, if possible. Comatose patients should also be given IV narcan, thiamine, and IV dextrose (if serum blood glucose levels cannot be determined) according to local protocols. Many elder patients with myxedema coma ultimately need mechanical ventilatory assistance. In-hospital treatment of patients with myxedema coma includes large doses of thyroxine. The expected mortality with adequate therapy still remains around 25 percent.

ADDISONIAN CRISIS

Addison's disease is the result of a failure of the adrenal glands to produce adequate amounts of cortisol. Addison's disease can present in elder patients with acute hypotension, abdominal pain, and confusion. Persons with Addison's disease may have hyperpigmentation in the creases of their palms, over their elbows, and on the insides of their cheeks. Addison's disease can result in severe hyperkalemia (increased blood potassium), hyponatremia (decreased blood sodium), and hypoglycemia. Hyperkalemia can cause unstable cardiac rhythms and shock. Stabilization in the prehospital setting involves the administration of intravenous saline, careful monitoring for shock, and administration of supplemental oxygen. In the confused patient, finding a medication bottle containing cortisol or prednisone in the home can be extremely helpful in making the diagnosis. If found, these bottles should be brought to the hospital for examination by hospital personnel.

REVIEW QUESTIONS

1. All of the following are true of type I diabetes *except*
   a. onset is usually age less than 30 years
   b. severe insulin deficiency
   c. usually requires treatment with insulin
   d. more common than type 2 diabetes in the elder population

2. All of the following are true of type 2 diabetes *except*
   a. usually ketosis and acidosis are absent
   b. onset age older than 40 years
   c. severe insulin deficiency
   d. often responds to oral hypoglycemics

3. Patients with acute onset of hyperglycemia have polyphagia because
   a. increased glucose levels stimulate the desire to eat
   b. increased insulin levels stimulate the desire to eat
   c. eating large amounts stimulates more insulin secretion
   d. glucose is lost in the urine, resulting in weight loss and the need to replace wasted glucose

4. When insulin deficiency is severe, the liver breaks fats down into
   a. ketones
   b. glucose
   c. proteins
   d. insulin

5. You respond to the home of a 70-year-old man who receives insulin through an insulin pump. He is extremely lethargic. His son states he has been ill and vomiting for 3 days. After initial ABCs and placement of an IV, a fingerstick blood sugar is >500 mg/dl. He has Kussmaul respirations, and his mouth and lips are dry. You suspect this man is suffering from
   a. hyperosmolar hyperglycemic non-ketotic coma
   b. diabetic ketoacidosis
   c. hypothyroidism
   d. hypoglycemic coma

6. In the patient in question 5, after administration of supplemental oxygen and cardiac monitoring, the most important prehospital therapy to initiate is
   a. IV insulin
   b. IV D50W
   c. IV normal saline bolus
   d. IV sodium bicarbonate

7. Care must be taken when giving IV normal saline to an elder patient in hyperosmolar hyperglycemic non-ketotic coma who also has a history of
   a. seizure disorder
   b. CVA
   c. coronary artery bypass graft
   d. congestive heart failure

8. Elder patients who are unresponsive in hypoglycemic coma (insulin shock) and have no IV access should be given
   a. oral glucose preparations
   b. D50W IM
   c. glucagon 10 mg IM
   d. glucagon 1 mg IM

9. All are features of thyrotoxicosis in the elder patient *except*
   a. cold intolerance
   b. weight loss
   c. atrial fibrillation
   d. congestive heart failure

10. Addison's disease in an elder patient can result in all of the following *except*
    a. hyponatremia
    b. hyperkalemia
    c. hypertension
    d. hypoglycemia

SUGGESTED READING

Harwood-Nuss, A., ed. 1996. *The clinical practice of emergency medicine,* 2d ed. Philadelphia: Lippincott–Raven.

Rosen, P. and Barkin, R., eds. 1998. *Emergency medicine. Concepts and clinical practice.* 4th ed. New York: Mosby.

9

Toxicologic Emergencies

Jonathan H. Valente, MD, and David C. Lee, MD

OBJECTIVES

By the end of this chapter, the prehospital health care provider should be able to:

1 Identify the presenting signs and symptoms of the major classes of toxic and drug exposures likely to be encountered in elders.

2 Discuss and carry out an initial and focused assessment of the patient with a toxic exposure.

3 Stabilize and transport these patients safely to appropriate secondary or tertiary care facilities.

CASE

You respond to a private home for an unknown medical emergency. On arrival, a woman tells you that her husband "passed out" in his chair in the living room. The patient is still sitting in his chair, conscious and mildly diaphoretic. He denies any pain and tells you he has been lightheaded all morning. He has had intermittent vomiting and diarrhea for the past 2 days. His vitals are: blood pressure 85/42, heart rate 40, respiratory rate 24. His wife tells you that he became unresponsive in his chair for 2 minutes, but did not have any seizure activity. She also states that he has a history of "heart trouble" and takes medication. As you place the patient on supplemental oxygen, start an IV of normal saline and begin cardiac monitoring, she hands you his medication list. The monitor shows that the patient is in third degree heart block. His medication list includes digoxin, hydrochlorothiazide, potassium, and a cholesterol lowering agent. What do you think is the problem with this man? What additional questions should you ask the patient or his wife? Is he in danger? What additional treatment can you offer him? Are there any medications you should consider giving him? If so, what are the appropriate dosages?

Toxic exposures in the form of drug overdoses, toxic inhalations, adverse drug reactions, and drug–drug interactions are common medical emergencies encountered in the United States. They account for approximately 4–5 million cases per year, with nearly 2 million cases reported to the American Association of Poison Centers Toxic Exposure Surveillance System (AAPCTESS). About 8 percent of these exposures involve patients older than 65. Both accidental as well as intentional ingestions are included. Kroner reported in 1993 that 84 percent of all exposures in elders were unintentional. Routes of exposure for toxic exposures include ingestions, inhalations, and splash ocular and dermal exposures. Onset and types of signs and symptoms vary according to the exposure. Often, the toxin or drug is not known, and the patient must be treated based solely on physical signs and symptoms. To assist with the medical management of such cases, Poison Control Centers are available to provide information to prehospital health care providers, doctors, nurses, and laypersons. These centers are available 24 hr a day and serve specific regions across the United States. All medical workers should be familiar with accessing their regional Poison Control Center. With cellular communication, a poison center should be available to most U.S. prehospital providers in the field.

ETIOLOGIES

The elder population is one of the most vulnerable to poisonings. Compared to adults under the age of 65, the elder patient, like the pediatric patient, is much more susceptible to subtle changes affecting different organ systems. Smaller ingestions or exposures have a greater potential to produce significant side effects or toxicities, more devastating consequences, and poorer outcomes. The geriatric population accounts for 8 percent of all exposures, yet they suffer 15 percent of all fatalities. Their higher morbidity and mortality rates are multifactorial.

Elders have greater exposure to potent pharmaceuticals. They consume approximately 30 percent of all prescribed medications, and 70 percent of elders use over-the-counter medications as well. Patients often receive multiple prescriptions from different health care professionals who do not communicate appropriately with each other, thus increasing the potential for adverse drug or drug–drug reactions. Elders often self-prescribe and borrow medications from other elders. New drugs are commonly tested only in younger patients prior to marketing. Many adverse reactions are discovered only after new drugs are distributed to the elder population.

Adverse drug reactions may be related to almost any complaint in elders. Depression, confusion, constipation, incontinence, urinary retention, and tremors are often interpreted as "normal" signs of aging, when in fact they may often be related to side effects of medications. Other common adverse drug effects may include mental status changes, dementia, and delirium. Acute delirium is a common presentation of drug toxicity in elders. Drugs well known to cause a change in mental status include anticholinergics (tricyclic antidepressants, antipsychotics, antihistamines, antiarrhythmics, ophthalmic preparations, antispasmodics, anticonvulsants, antiparkinsonians, over-the-counter sleep/allergy medications), sedative/hypnotics, steroids, H2 blockers, dopaminergic agents, and digoxin. In 1989, the U.S. Food and Drug Administration (FDA) released guidelines encouraging involvement of elder subjects in drug development and marketing specifically to uncover adverse drug reactions in elders as efficiently as possible.

Social and environmental factors often can precipitate inadvertent poisonings in elders. Unintentional poisonings often result from failure to understand instructions or read labels because of confusion, disorientation, diminishing cognitive capacity or, simply, poor vision. Other examples of social and environmental factors that lead to drug ingestion errors include inability to organize drug storage containers or medicine cabinets, poor lighting in the elder's home, lack of proper compliance with prescribed medications, and socioeconomic factors such as borrowing or sharing medications because of poverty.

The risk of fatal intentional exposures increases with age. Suicide among elders is a common cause of death, being highest among white males. Drug overdoses, including toxic inhalations, are the most common method of suicide among elder females. Depression and alcoholism are common and frequently underdiagnosed in elders. Thus, a high index of suspicion and a thorough investigation must be sought in all cases in which signs and symptoms suggest an intentional overdose.

The aging process causes physiological changes that render the elder patient more susceptible to adverse drug effects. Processes within the body, such as absorption, metabolism, and elimination of drugs and toxins, function less efficiently as the human body ages. Both kidney and liver function diminish with age, and both organs are involved in properly eliminating different drugs and toxins. The kidney's glomerular filtration rate decreases by 35–50 percent, leading to a reduction in clearance of certain drugs. Commonly, there is a decrease in blood flow to the liver, causing impaired metabolism and excretion of drugs. Elders also have lower total body water content, lower volume of distribution of water-soluble drugs, and lower lean muscle mass, which can alter the distribution of drugs within the tissues of the body. They have greater (potentially toxic) systemic drug concentration at what would be a therapeutic drug dose in a younger patient. Homeostasis is not as well maintained in elders. Heart rate and blood pressure do not respond as rapidly to compensate for toxic stresses.

Common adverse drug and toxin reactions are listed in Table 9.1.

Table 9.1. Common Adverse Drug and Toxin Reactions

Altered Mental Status
Opioids/sedatives/hypnotics
Anticholinergics (antihistamines, antiparkinsonians, atropine, antipsychotics, antidepressants, anticonvulsants, antispasmodics/muscle relaxants)
Theophylline
Digoxin
Isoniazid (INH)
Cholinergics (insecticides)
Alcohols
Carbon monoxide
Methemoglobinemia (acetanilid, aniline dyes, chlorates, nitrites)
Withdrawal (alcohol, benzodiazepines, barbiturates, opioids)
Heavy metals (rare)
Tricyclic antidepressants (TCAs)
Lithium
Hypoxia as a result of inhalation of butane, propane, methane, carbon dioxide (displaces oxygen)
See also hypoglycemia list

(continued)

Table 9.1. Continued

Seizures[a]
  Amphetamines (5)
  INH (3)
  Theophylline (4)
  Lithium
  Tricyclic antidepressants (TCAs) (1)
  Over-the-counter decongestants
  Cocaine (2)
  Carbon monoxide
  Methemoglobinemia
  Anticholinergics
  Cholinergics
  Withdrawal

Hypotension/Syncope
  Nitroglycerin (nitrates)
  Opioids
  Calcium-channel blockers
  Beta-blockers
  ACE inhibitors
  Diuretics
  See also arrhythmias list

Arrhythmias/Syncope
  Antiarrhythmics (quinidine, procainamide)
  Digoxin
  Cocaine
  Amphetamines
  Theophylline
  TCAs
  Synthroid
  Over-the-counter decongestants
  Lithium
  Erythromycin
  Anti-seizure medications (phenytoin)

Hypoglycemia
  Insulin
  Oral hypoglycemics
  Alcohol, salicylates, and beta-blockers (as a result of the
    underproduction of glucose)
  INH

[a]The five most common causes of drug-induced seizures secondary to overdose are indicated in the table.

ASSESSMENT

Safety and Decontamination

Exposures to toxins may occur in several ways, including ingestions, inhalations, dermal absorptions, and injections. The potential presence of hazardous materials in the environment in a prehospital response to a toxic exposure demands that scene safety be a very important aspect of prehospital emergency care. In order to minimize exposure to health care workers, the scene must be quickly and thoroughly investigated for potential continued poison exposure to both the patient and the rescue workers. For example, the elder patient found in a burning building, automobile, garage, or home with a wood-burning stove must be moved quickly from the potentially dangerous scene to an open air environment. Such patients may have been exposed to carbon monoxide or cyanide gases. In addition, rescue workers should wear appropriate protective equipment as needed (e.g., masks, gloves) and enter sites only in areas where training and expertise allow safe entry. If unsure about scene safety, do not rush into a scene until protective equipment is available or the HAZMAT team has cleared the scene. Patients with chemical exposure to their skin and clothes such as insecticides or corrosives may continue to be exposed or expose rescuers unless appropriate decontamination protocols are instituted. Decontamination procedures may include removing the patient from the scene, removing the patient's clothes and jewelry, and irrigating the skin with copious amounts of water for 20–30 min to remove wet chemicals or brushing off dry chemicals from skin surfaces. Always attempt to decontaminate the airway and face first, if possible. For eye exposures, irrigation with 1–2 liters of normal saline should begin immediately.

A variety of decontamination methods exist for treating the elder patient with a poison ingestion. Two are of particular importance to the prehospital health care provider. The first, activated charcoal, possesses a large surface area for binding ingested particles of certain drugs and other substances to decrease absorption. The second, ipecac, is used to induce vomiting. Although ipecac is still standard issue on most rescue vehicles and ambulances, it is no longer recommended as a routine treatment for toxic ingestions in elders, especially when transport times are less than 1 hr. Ipecac can cause continued vomiting on reaching the hospital, making it difficult to administer activated charcoal and specific antidotes to the patient. In addition, elder patients given ipecac who have a decreased level of consciousness from the ingestion or from a previous neurological problem and have a deficient gag reflex are at serious risk for aspiration with vomiting. Activated charcoal has been shown to be as effective as ipecac or stomach irrigation (gastric lavage). Gastric lavage is performed in the emergency department using a large-bore tube passed to the stomach through the mouth to physically decontaminate the poisoned patient. It can pose a risk to the patient, and the decision to lavage rests with the emergency medicine specialist. Activated charcoal has been shown to work better when given soon after ingestion and has been recommended in prehospital protocols for ingestions in the awake elder patient during transport, especially during longer transports. However, activated charcoal has *not* been shown to be useful in ingestions of hydrocarbons, acid–alkali substances, alcohols, or heavy metals such as lead, iron, and mercury. If in doubt about whether to use activated charcoal in the elder patient with a toxic ingestion, refer to local protocols or consult the on-line medical control physician.

History

Often the history of exposure in the elder poisoned patient is unreliable. The patient may have altered mental status or may refuse to cooperate (intentional ingestions). However, always make every attempt to obtain a complete history at the scene. The information obtined by the prehospital health care provider may be the only data that the emergency department staff has to work with. Make every effort to identify the toxin, drug, chemical, or gas. Search for clues or evidence at the scene, including odors, bottles, pills on the floor, vomitus, bystander information, suicide notes, space heaters, or rooms adjacent to garage doors. Take any evidence with you to the hospital. Try to determine when the exposure occurred and how much of the substance was ingested. Attempt to estimate volume of exposure (i.e., how much chemical remaining in the bottle). Find out how the patient was exposed and for how long. Record the patient's symptoms. Ask the patient about suicide attempts in the present or past. Never forget to consider trauma in the elder patient that has occurred after a poison exposure. Keep in mind that elders are more likely to have toxic substances in their homes that have been there for many years, and may no longer be available for sale. These substances (e.g., insecticides) may be unfamiliar to the prehospital health care provider as well as emergency department personnel. Thus it cannot be overemphasized that careful scene assessment to identify possible toxins that an elder patient might have come into contact with can be life saving.

A simple pneumonic provides a SAMPLE history. This refers to Signs and symptoms, Allergies, Medications, Past medical/surgical history, Last meal the patient ate, and Event data surrounding the present condition. Thoroughly evaluate the patient's environment. Gather any evidence that may be helpful in the treatment of the patient. This may include any pills or pill bottles, containers, and suicide notes. As many elder patients are still in the workforce, Material Safety Data Sheets (MSDS) may also be available.

RETURNING TO THE CASE

The patient is suffering from digitalis toxicity. You learn from his wife that the patient takes his medications on his own, but sometimes gets confused. She thinks he may not be taking the correct medicines or in the correct dosages. You administer atropine, 1 mg IV, with no change in the patient's heart rate or rhythm. A repeat dose of atropine is also ineffective. You then place the patient on an external pacemaker and his heart rate increases to your set rate of 80 beats per minute (bpm) with 100% capture. His blood pressure improves to 110/70. Aside from some mild discomfort associated with the pacemaker, he feels improved. You transport him rapidly to the emergency department.

Any elder patient exhibiting altered mental status, seizure, syncope, hypotension, arrhythmia, or hypoglycemia may have an intentional drug overdose, an adverse drug reaction, a drug–drug interaction, or an inhalation. Take a careful history of medications, including over-the counter drugs and any recent medication changes. Often a medication list is available and should be brought with the patient to the emergency department.

Initial assessment as always starts with the ABCs (Airway, Breathing, Circulation). On focused assessment, after the vital signs and cardiovascular and respiratory systems, evaluate the patient's mental status and perform a neurological exam. The AVPU system is an easy and highly reproducible evaluation of the patient's mental status: spontaneously Alert, responding to Verbal stimuli, responding to Painful stimuli, and Unresponsive. Another well-studied and reproducible mental status evaluation is the Glasgow Coma Scale. Look for any evidence of trauma, including head trauma, cervical spine injury, burns, stab wounds, and bullet holes. After these patients have been initially evaluated, they must be continually reassessed and reevaluated enroute to the hospital.

Stabilization and Treatment

Although the etiology and presentation of toxic exposure in the elder patient is different from that of the younger patient, the prehospital stabilization and management of toxic exposure in the elder patient is similar to that of younger patients.

If the elder patient with a toxic exposure is breathing, administer 100 percent oxygen via nonrebreather mask. If the patient is not breathing, establish a patent airway and provide positive pressure ventilation with 100 percent O_2 via bag–valve mask. If the patient is unconscious or cannot protect their airway, a secure airway should be established with endotracheal intubation. Establish IV access with normal saline or lactated ringer's solution and draw blood for glucose. If possible, check fingerstick glucose. Establish cardiac monitoring of the patient. If the patient is hypoglycemic or if unable to determine this status, then give 100 mg thiamine IV plus D50 (25 g dextrose–50 cc of 50 percent solution). If you are unable to establish an IV, give glucagon 1 mg IM to patients with suspected hypoglycemia. (Note: If the patient is awake with an adequate gag response and able to drink unassisted, it is permissible to give oral glucose solution.) Reassess the patient. For elder patients with altered mental status or unconsciousness, if there is no change, give naloxone (Narcan®) 2 mg IV. Naloxone may also be administered IM or via ET tube depending on regional protocols. Repeat doses of D50 or naloxone (maximum dose is 10 mg) may be given if there is no response in mental status or respiratory rate. Transport the patient to the hospital.

Hypotension as a result of drug ingestion generally results from vascular decompensation or cardiac malfunction. Crystalloid fluids such as normal saline and lactated ringer's provide good initial volume support. However, if blood pressures continue to remain low in a symptomatic patient, vasopressors such as dopamine and norepinephrine may be considered.

Ventilatory support with 100 percent oxygen is required for all suspected carbon monoxide or inhalation exposures. Bronchodilators are indicated in the wheezing patient after pulmonary irritant inhalations. In some overdoses, specific treatments are required that deviate from the standard American Cardiac Life Support (ACLS) guidelines. Patients with tricyclic antidepressant overdoses may manifest a wide complex tachycardia associated with hypotension that is often resistant to standard ACLS therapy. In such cases, crystalloids and intravenous sodium bicarbonate followed by norepinephrine provide a much better response. In tricyclic antidepressant overdoses, dopamine causes unopposed peripheral beta-receptor effects (vasodilatation of arteries and artieroles), leading to worsening hypotension. Patients with calcium channel blocker overdoses may have a bradycardia associated with hypotension. Intravenous calcium (CaCl 1 g IV push) or calcium gluconate (3 g) may be given for hypotension. Other common overdoses causing hemodynamic instability in the elder patient include digoxin and beta-blockers. Treatments such as atropine and external cardiac pacing are indicated for symptomatic bradydysrhythmias. Lidocaine is indicated for ventricular dysrhythmias. Glucagon (1 mg IM) can be used in refractory cases of beta-blocker or calcium channel blocker overdose. In addition, specific treatments such as Fab fragments (Digibind®) may be ordered by the poison center or physician on-line for medical control. Digibind® is indicated for digoxin overdose with life-threatening dysrhythmias. For specific toxic ingestions in which resuscitation deviates from established protocols, always rely on physician and base station control if available.

> ## CASE OUTCOME
>
> In the emergency department, the patient is maintained on the external pacemaker during his work-up and remains stable. He is found to have an elevated serum digoxin level and low potassium (which was felt to have worsened the digoxin toxicity). He was given Fab fragments (Digibind®) and potassium replacement, and in a few hours returned to a normal sinus rhythm. He was discharged home 2 days later, and agreed that his wife should dispense his medications.

CONCLUSION

Elders experiencing a toxic exposure, ingestion, inhalation, drug reaction or interaction may present in subtle or atypical ways. Always maintain a high index of suspicion when elders present with unusual signs and symptoms. Always maintain scene safety. Treat the patient symptomatically adhering to the ABC's and stabilizing, gather data carefully from the scene and any exposure information that you can, obtain a good medical history, and transport rapidly to the appropriate hospital while frequently reassessing the patient.

REVIEW QUESTIONS

1. Toxic exposures in elders include all of the following *except*
   a. drug–drug interactions
   b. inhalations
   c. adverse drug reactions
   d. anaphylactic reactions

2. Which of the following is *true* regarding toxic exposures in elders?
   a. Approximately 50 percent of all overdoses in the United States occur in elders.
   b. Most toxic exposures in elders are unintentional.
   c. The type of toxic exposure is usually known to prehospital personnel.
   d. Elders manifest the same signs and symptoms as the younger population.

3. Poison Control Centers should only be contacted by
   a. patients
   b. prehospital health care providers
   c. hospital based nurses or physicians
   d. all of the above

4. Elders have greater potential for adverse drug reactions and drug–drug interactions because of all of the following *except*
   a. elders consume 30 percent of all medications prescribed in the United States
   b. elders frequently share medications
   c. elders frequently take their medications all at once or not at all
   d. elders often have multiple physicians, and often receive medications from each one

5. Drugs commonly associated with changes in mental status in elders include all of the following *except*
   a. antihypertensives
   b. antipsychotics
   c. antihistamines
   d. anticholinergics

6. Elders are more susceptible than young people to drug toxicities because of all of the following *except*
   a. absorbtion of drugs is less efficient
   b. metabolism of drugs is slower
   c. neurologic processing is less efficient
   d. elimination of drugs is less efficient

7. Activated charcoal can be administered safely in the prehospital setting to elder patients with toxic exposures
   a. only after syrup of ipecac has been administered
   b. to awake patients during long transports
   c. resulting from hyrocarbon ingestion
   d. only after 3 hr have passed since the ingestion

8. Appropriate scene assessment includes all of the following *except*
   a. leaving all unknown toxins at the scene, as they may be dangerous
   b. searching for clues at the scene and reporting them to hospital personnel
   c. evaluating the patient for possible traumatic injuries related to the toxic exposure
   d. attempting to determine the time of exposure and the length of exposure

9. Match the exposure or adverse reaction with the appropriate treatment
   a. hypoglycemia   bronchodilators
   b. narcotic overdose   Fab fragments
   c. digitalis toxicity   glucagon
   d. pulmonary irritant inhalations   calcium chloride
   e. calcium channel blocker overdose   naloxone

10. In severe tricyclic antidepressant overdose, administration of dopamine can cause
   a. normalization of blood pressure
   b. ventricular tachycardia
   c. change in mental status
   d. hypotension

SUGGESTED READING

Cassel, C. K. 1997. *Geriatric medicine*. New York: Springer-Verlag, Inc., pp. 55–67.

Crockett, R. 1996. Prehospital use of activated charcoal: A pilot study. *The Journal of Emergency Medicine* 14:335–338.

Ellenhorn, M. J. 1997. *Ellenhorn's medical toxicology: Diagnosis and treatment of human poisoning*. Baltimore: Williams & Wilkins, a Waverly Company, pp. 128–144.

Goldfrank, L. R. 1994. *Goldfrank's toxicologic emergencies*. Norwalk, CT: Appleton & Lange, pp. 447–453.

Gonzalez, D. 1996. *Prehospital advanced life support protocols*. The Regional EMS Council of NYC, Inc.

Harwood-Nuss, A. 1991. *The clinical practice of emergency medicine*. Philadelphia: J. B. Lippincott Co., pp. 430–442.

Kroner, B. A., R. B. Scott, E. R. Waring, and J. R. Zanga. 1993. Poisoning in the elderly: Characterization of exposures reported to a poison control center. *Journal of the American Geriatric Society* 41:842–846.

Markovchick, V. J. 1993. *Emergency medicine secrets*. Philadelphia: Hanley and Belfus, Inc., pp. 283–288.

Paramedic Protocols. 1995. *Naussau regional EMS advanced life support protocol and policy manual,* Section III.

Tintinalli, J. E. 1996. *Emergency medicine: A comprehensive study guide*. New York: The McGraw-Hill Companies, Inc., pp. 735–740.

10

Environmental Emergencies

Robert Partridge, MD, MPH

OBJECTIVES

This chapter focuses on environmental emergencies frequently encountered by the elder population. By the end of this chapter, the prehospital health care professional should be able to:

1 Recognize and define hypothermia.
2 Stabilize and treat an elder patient with hypothermia.
3 Define heat stroke, heat exhaustion, and heat syncope.
4 Stabilize and treat an elder patient with heat illness.
5 Recognize and describe thermal burns.
6 Stabilize an elder patient with thermal burns.

CASE

You respond to the home of an elder man with an unknown emergency. It is mid-July and the outside temperature is 38.8°C (102°F). The patient's apartment is on the top floor of a nine-story building, and the temperature inside is even warmer. You are let into the apartment by the patient's wife, who directs you to a rear bedroom. As you survey the scene, you see that the only cooling device in the apartment is a small table fan. The patient is lying in bed with the bedclothes over him. He is awake but obviously confused. On initial assessment, his respiratory rate is 28, pulse is 120, blood pressure is 160/90, and his skin is hot and dry. On focused assessment he is completely disoriented and hallucinating, but is able to move all four extremities. There is no evidence of trauma. His wife hands you a bag of medications and you find some cardiac and some antipsychotic medications. What do you think is the problem with this man? What additional history should you ask for? How sick is he? Is he in danger? What prehospital stabilization and treatment should you initiate prior to hospital transfer? What about the patient's wife? If she refuses to go to the hospital, should you intervene for her safety?

HYPOTHERMIA AND HEAT ILLNESS

A person's ability to regulate temperature declines with increasing age. Elder persons are less able to control body temperature when exposed to extremes of environmental temperature. Hypothermia and hyperthermia are most common in the elder population. Both morbidity and mortality of the elder population increases during environmental extremes of temperature, especially among elder persons who are already ill. Elder persons are more likely to suffer myocardial infarction, stroke, and pneumonia as a result of hypothermia and hyperthermia.

Hypothermia

Hypothermia in the elder population is more common in the winter months in northern climates. Studies have shown that as many as 10 percent of elder people living at home are borderline hypothermic, with core temperatures below 35.5°C (95.9°F), and that as many as 3.6 percent of all patients older than 65 admitted to the hospital are hypothermic. However, it is important to remember that hypothermia in the elder population can occur in any climate and any season, depending on environmental conditions.

Etiology. *Hypothermia* is defined as a core temperature of less than 35°C (95°F). Environmental mechanisms of heat loss result from conduction (direct contact with a cooler object), convection (cooling as a result of air movement around the body, such as wind), evaporation (heat lost with evaporating moisture from the skin), and radiation (direct loss of electromagnetic heat energy to the environment). When exposed to environmental conditions that can result in hypothermia, elder persons are more susceptible to hypothermia because of underlying disease processes and physiologic changes associated with aging. The thermoregulatory center controls body temperature through a variety of mechanisms, including sweating, vasoconstriction and vasodilation, chemical production of heat, and shivering. Elder persons have impaired sensitivity to cold and changes in ambient temperature. Elders have impaired shivering and vasoconstrictor response to the cold, as well as poorer heat production. Thin elder persons are also at risk because of reduced insulation.

Certain disease processes common in the elder population predispose this group to hypothermia. These include hypothyroidism, hypoglycemia, starvation, and malnutrition. Any insult to the cerebral thermoregulatory system can contribute to hypothermia in elders, including trauma, hypoxia, tumor, or cerebrovascular disease. Alcohol and certain drugs, including barbiturates, phenothiazines, benzodiazepines, and narcotics, all can increase the risk of hypothermia for an elder patient. Hypothermia in elders also occurs in sepsis (infection that overwhelms host defenses) and with underlying cardiovascular disease because the circulatory system cannot respond to the demands required to shiver.

Finally, socioeconomic factors can also predispose the elder population. Many elders live alone and may not have central heating or, because of dementia or confusion, may fail to use it.

Assessment. For the reasons already listed, it is imperative that the prehospital health care provider consider hypothermia in any elder patient exposed to environmental conditions that cause heat loss. Remember that hypothermia can occur in any season in any climate in the appropriate environmental conditions. Although in the elder population hypothermia is more common in winter, prolonged exposure to wind and rain on a cool summer day can also cause hypothermia in an elder patient.

A diagnosis of hypothermia can be recognized only with a low-reading thermometer, which may not be standard equipment on all ambulances, depending on local protocols. *Mild hypothermia* is defined as a core temperature of 32–35°C (89.6–95°F). Because clinical signs are subtle in mild hypothermia, a high index of suspicion is mandatory so that this diagnosis is not missed. In mild hypothermia, an elder patient may complain of cold, fatigue, or weakness; they may have an impaired gait, apathy, slurred speech, confusion, and cool skin or shivering.

Moderate hypothermia is defined as a core temperature of 28–32°C (82.4–89.6°F), and clinical symptoms are more pronounced. The skin is cold, and patients are semiconscious or unconscious, with shallow respirations, cyanosis, and bradycardia. Muscular rigidity may also be present. Ventricular arrhythmias and hypotension (shock) may occur.

Severe hypothermia occurs when the core temperature drops below 28°C (82.4°F). In this clinical condition, the elder patient is unresponsive, with complete muscular rigidity. The pupils may be fixed and dilated, and the patient may be apneic. Ventricular fibrillation occurs in severe hypothermia, and is seen on the cardiac monitor. The PR, QRS, and QT intervals may also be prolonged. Another electrocardiographic abnormality that may be seen on the monitor is the J wave (also called the *Osborn wave*). The J wave looks like an upgoing notch and immediately follows the QRS complex. As the patient is rewarmed, the J wave disappears.

In severe hypothermia, the skin is extremely cold and the patient may appear to have been dead for several hours. However, there are many recorded instances of a patient being successfully rewarmed and resuscitated after being found hypothermic and apparently dead, so always remember that when assessing an elder hypothermic patient that they should never be considered dead until they have been thoroughly rewarmed. Transfer of such patients to a hospital emergency department, preferably a hospital capable of rapid core rewarming with cardiac bypass, is always indicated.

Stabilization and treatment. In the prehospital setting, treatment depends on the degree of hypothermia. After a quick initial assessment of airway, breathing, and circulation (ABCs), the elder patient with hypothermia should be immediately removed from the cold environment, wind, and contact with cold objects. Remember to stabilize the cervical spine prior to moving the patient if trauma is suspected. All wet clothing should be removed. Peripheral intravenous access should be established, the patient should be placed on the cardiac monitor, and supplemental oxygen should be administered. Intermittent suctioning of airway secretions may be required. The ambulance should be prewarmed and, if possible, blankets should be prewarmed. Warm blankets should be placed both over and under the patient. Every effort should be made to ensure that the patient is moved carefully, without any sudden jolts or movements. A complete medication list should be brought with the patient to the receiving facility.

The myocardium of a hypothermic patient is extremely irritable, and any sudden movement may cause ventricular fibrillation. Any hypothermic patient who has a detectable pulse and any respiratory effort should not receive chest compressions, endotracheal intubation, or unnecessary movements needed to place a temporary pacemaker. Ventilations can be gently assisted with an ambu-bag. Intravenous fluids should be initiated and prewarmed, if possible. If an elder patient is asystolic or in ventricular fibrillation, he or she should be resuscitated. The cold heart is usually unresponsive to defibrillation and drugs. Although core temperature should be at least 32°C (89.6°F) prior to attempts at ventricular defibrillation, it is often not possible to correctly ascertain the core temperature in the prehospital setting. Therefore, if ventricular fibrillation is present, it is permissible to attempt cardiac defibrillation *once*, as further attempts will likely be unsuccessful and cause further irritation to the myocardium. If initial defibrillation is unsuccessful, continue with standard ACLS protocols without further attempts at defibrillation.

Elder patients with any degree of hypothermia should be transferred immediately to a hospital emergency department for further rewarming and treatment. If severe hypothermia is present, transfer to a facility capable of rapid core rewarming with cardiac bypass or continuous arteriovenous rewarming is preferable.

RETURNING TO THE CASE

This man is suffering from heat stroke. He is hyperthermic, confused, hallucinating, and his skin is hot—he is not perspiring to lower his body temperature. He is critically ill, and he is at higher risk of mortality from this illness because he is taking some anticholinergic medications. You place him on oxygen and the cardiac monitor, which shows a sinus tachycardia, and quickly move him to your air-conditioned vehicle. You establish an IV with normal saline and give a 500 cc fluid bolus. You pack his axillae, groins, and carotid areas with ice packs and transport him to the hospital, along with his wife.

HEAT ILLNESS

Heat illness typically occurs in warmer climates, especially during heat waves. There are about 5000 deaths annually in the United States as a consequence of hyperthermia, approximately two-thirds of which are in the elder population, and may be related to the fact that hyperthermia can increase cardiovascular morbidity and mortality in elders.

Hyperthermia can be divided into several important clinical syndromes. *Heat stroke* is a sudden failure of the body to maintain a constant normal temperature in a warm environment. Heat stroke is an acute life-threatening emergency that results in the elevation of body temperature to extreme levels, often greater than

41°C (106°F), and causes multiple organ system failure. Heat stroke is most commonly seen in the elder population. *Heat exhaustion* is a condition of fluid or electrolyte depletion that occurs during heat stress. This condition frequently results from inadequate fluid intake by persons exerting themselves in a hot environment, such as laborers, athletes, and other individuals who have no access to fluids in a hot environment. If untreated, heat exhaustion can progress to heat stroke. *Heat syncope* is a condition characterized by sudden and transient loss of consciousness in a hot environment. It is believed to be related to sudden dilation of peripheral blood vessels to radiate heat from the skin, but causes transient intravascular hypotension and syncope. Heat syncope is most often seen in elders, because they are more likely to have underlying cardiovascular disease or may be on medications that may contribute to syncope.

Etiology. Elder persons are more prone to heat illness than younger populations for several reasons. Elders may have dysfunction of the heat regulating center in the brain, and may also have a diminished ability to sweat. Some elders may also have delayed vasodilation of the skin in response to a hot environment. Older individuals may have impaired sensitivity to temperature changes, which can result in inappropriate adaptive behaviors when exposed to a hot environment. Living alone, immobility, and confusion can also cause elder persons to take inadequate cooling measures in a hot environment. For example, elders may not remove heavy clothing, move inside or to a cooler environment, turn on air conditioners or fans, or call for help. Elders on fixed incomes may delay or avoid using air conditioners because of increased electrical costs. Congestive heart failure, diabetes mellitus, obesity, and emphysema, all common conditions in elders, are risk factors for death in elders with heat illness. Other factors that increase mortality in heat illness are alcoholism and use of sedatives and anticholinergic medications. Anticholinergics, including phenothiazines and antidepressants, can contribute to impaired sweating and worsen heat illness. Diuretics may cause hypovolemia, and beta-blockers may contribute to impaired myocardial function, both of which can worsen heat illness.

Assessment. Heat stroke in elders is characterized by a temperature of greater than 40.6°C (105°F) during exposure to a hot environment; severe central nervous system dysfunction, including psychosis, delirium, seizures, or coma; and hot, dry skin. The prehospital health care provider should be particularly mindful of heat stroke in the elder population during heat waves. It is also important for the prehospital health care provider to remember that heat stroke can also occur after a period of heavy exertion, when the body is producing excess heat that becomes improperly regulated, and that heat stroke can occur at body temperatures as low as 39.5°C (103°F). In 80 percent of patients the onset of heat stroke is sudden, and the patient rapidly progresses to delirium and coma. In about 20 percent of cases elder patients initially have nonspecific symptoms, including weakness, dizziness, nausea, vomiting, headache, confusion, drowsiness, disorientation, muscle twitching, and difficulty with balance and irritability. Many of these initial features may be seen in heat exhaustion. Although patients may initially have normal blood pressure, if they are hypovolemic or if heat stroke is advanced, they may be in shock. Numerous cardiac arrythmias may be seen on the monitor.

Heat exhaustion is characterized by a body temperature that may be normal or elevated, but usually not greater than 39°C (102.2°F). Central nervous system function is normal—seizures and coma are *not* present. Elder patients with heat exhaustion may complain of vague symptoms such as malaise, fatigue, muscle cramps, and headache. Tachycardia, orthostatic hypotension, and clinical dehydration may be present. In heat exhaustion, sweating persists, and the skin is diaphoretic. It is important that prehospital health care provider assessing an elder patient with signs of heat exhaustion in a hot environment realize that heat exhaustion can rapidly progress to heat stroke, so removal from the environment, stabilization, and transport must occur without delay.

Heat syncope is characterized by transient syncope when exposed to a hot environment and is more common in elders than in any other age group. The patient is usually awake at the time of prehospital health care provider arrival, and has a normal temperature, blood pressure, and pulse. Heat syncope is difficult to differentiate from syncope because of other causes in the prehospital setting. Placing a patient in the supine position is the cure, and patients should still be transferred to the emergency department for a complete syncope evaluation. In the prehospital setting, heat syncope should be treated like syncope from any other cause—patients should be placed on a cardiac monitor and supplemental oxygen provided; vital signs should be monitored, an intravenous line should be established, and a fingerstick glucose performed. A complete secondary survey to assess the patient for trauma should also be completed.

Stabilization and treatment. Initial treatment of elder patients with heat-related illness involves establishing and maintaining airway, breathing, and circulation. Administer supplemental oxygen and place the patient on a cardiac monitor. Establish large bore (18-gauge needle or greater) intravenous access. Patients who are unresponsive or who cannot protect their own airway should be intubated. A patient who is in shock should be given a bolus of normal saline (250–500 cc). Unstable arrhythmias should be treated according to usual arrhythmia protocols. Elder patients suffering from heat stroke require rapid cooling because longer duration of hyperthermia is associated with poorer outcome. Rapid cooling should begin in the field as soon as initial stabilization has been performed. The goal is to bring the body temperature down to 39°C (102.2°F) in the first hour of treatment. All heavy or unnecessary clothing should be removed immediately. Ice packs should be applied to the neck, armpits, and groins. Air-conditioning units should be turned on in the ambulance, and if possible, a cooling fan should be directed toward the patient to maximize convective heat loss. Alcohol sponge baths should *not* be used in the prehospital setting, because alcohol may be absorbed into the blood stream through dilated blood vessels in the skin and cause lethargy or coma. After initial stabilization and treatment, all elder patients with heat stroke should be transferred to the nearest receiving facility without delay.

Prehospital stabilization and treatment of the patient with suspected heat exhaustion is similar to that of heat stroke, except that the patient may not be profoundly hyperthermic, so rapid cooling may not be necessary. However, when in doubt or if no thermometer is available, and the patient is in a warm environment with mental status changes and hot, dry skin, always err on the side of treatment for heat stroke and initiate rapid cooling procedures.

As mentioned previously, it is difficult to differentiate heat syncope from syncope of other etiologies. Elder patients with suspected heat syncope should be stabilized and treated like any other syncope patient.

It is important for the prehospital health care provider to realize that the most effective strategy for reducing the incidence of hypothermia or heat-related illness in elders is prevention. Education of older patients about their risk and increased susceptibility to hypothermia or heat-related illness can be provided. Education can also focus on appropriate actions for an elder person to take if exposed to extremes of temperature. The most vulnerable elder patients (those with dementia, immobility, or limited resources) should be monitored closely to reduce their risk of morbidity or mortality. Finally, prehospital health care providers should remember that they may be the only health care provider an elder patient has who can assess the living conditions in the home and identify patients at risk for hypothermia, heat-related illness, and other potentially serious conditions. Any patient with an immediate health risk should be transferred to a health care facility for evaluation. Any patient with a significant potential for morbidity or mortality because of environmental causes should be reported to the appropriate state authorities, social services agency, or department of elder affairs.

THERMAL BURNS

Burn wounds can result from scalds, contact burns, fire, chemicals, electricity, and radiation. This section focuses on thermal burns as a result of scalds, contact burns, and fire. Elder patients actually have a lower incidence of burn injury than the remainder of the population. Those older than 80 years of age are least likely to sustain a serious burn injury (2.3 percent). In this age group, however, hot-surface exposure in particular is a major cause of thermal burns. Chemical and electrical burns are not frequently encountered in the elder population. The evaluation and management of liquid or solid chemical burns and electrical burns in elders in the prehospital setting does not differ from the general population.

Burn severity is related to the rate at which heat is transferred to the skin. This rate of transfer is dependent on the heat capacity of the burn agent, temperature of the agent, duration of contact, coefficient of heat transfer, and conductivity of local tissues. Heat capacity describes the amount of heat a material contains when it comes into contact with the skin. The quantity of heat stored in a material depends on the amount of energy required to heat it to a particular temperature. For example, the amount of heat required to heat water is more than 10 times that required to heat copper. Thus if both of these agents are at the same temperature and come into contact with the skin, the water transfers more than 10 times the amount of heat energy to the skin than copper. The initial temperature of the material at the moment of contact with the skin is an important factor in the severity of burn injury. The higher the temperature, the greater the amount of burn energy transferred to the skin. Duration of contact with the skin is important because if the temperature of the burning agent is greater than 40°C (104°F), the amount of tissue destruction increases dramatically as contact time increases. Duration of contact is particularly important with liquids. Liquids that are more viscous (thicker), like oils, tend to cling to the skin and worsen the burn injury. In immersion burns, or scalds, the duration of contact with the skin is longer than with splash or spill scalds.

Types of Burns

Burns are categorized according to the depth of tissue injury. A *first-degree burn* is a burn to the epidermis, or outermost layer, of skin. The skin is tender, red, and patients complain of pain. The skin is not blistered. A sunburn is a typical example.

A *second-degree burn* is defined as a burn of the epidermis and the dermis. The *dermis* is the living layer of skin beneath the epidermis, which contains capillaries, hair follicles, glands, and other supporting structures. A second-degree burn, depending on the depth, may have thin-walled or thick-walled blisters. A superficial second-degree burn blisters with thin walls, and if they have ruptured, the underlying skin appears pink and moist and is extremely tender to touch. More serious (deeper) second-degree burns have blisters with thicker walls that may not rupture spontaneously. The underlying skin in a deeper second-degree burn is red and in some places may be white. Sensation is diminished, but at the very least the patient should feel pressure on palpation of these burned areas. Second-degree burns are usually caused by steam or scalds.

A *third-degree burn* is a full thickness burn that causes destruction of the epidermis and the dermis and into the subcutaneous fat. Third-degree burns usually do not blister. The skin appears whitish and feels like leather. All sensation is absent. Third-degree burns are usually caused by prolonged scalds, flame, or high-voltage electricity.

Fourth-degree burns are full thickness burns that extend well into subcutaneous tissue and may involve connective tissue, muscle, or bone. These are very serious burns and result from prolonged exposure to agents that cause third-degree burns.

Assessment

A common and practical technique for assessing extent of burns is the "rule of nines." This method divides the body into percentages of total body surface area (BSA). In adults, the head and neck represent 9 percent BSA, the front and back of the torso 18 percent BSA each, the upper extremities 9 percent BSA each, and the lower extremities 18 percent BSA each. The genital area represents 1 percent BSA. Use the patient's palm to assess smaller areas of BSA—the palm equals about 1 percent BSA. Add up percentages of BSA from different areas to calculate a total BSA burn. Further subdivision of burns into total BSA of different degrees of burns (partial thickness and full thickness) is also helpful in making a full assessment.

The American Burn Association classifies burns into major, moderate, and minor burns. A *major burn* is a partial thickness burn of 25 percent BSA in adults or 20 percent BSA in adults older than 50 years of age; a full thickness burn of more than 10 percent BSA; burns of the face, eyes, ears, hands, feet, or perineum that may result in cosmetic or functional impairment; burns caused by caustic chemicals, high-voltage electricity; burns complicated by inhalation injury or major trauma; or burns in patients with other underlying disease, especially elders. Patients with major burn injuries are best served at a designated burn center. A *moderate burn* is a partial thickness burn of 15–25 percent BSA in adults, or 10–20 percent BSA in older adults and full thickness burns of 2–10 percent BSA not likely to cause functional or cosmetic impairment, and not involving the face, eyes, hands, feet, or perineum. Burns complicated by trauma, inhalation injury, or other underlying disease, or caused by caustic chemicals or high-voltage electricity, do not fall in this category. Patients with moderate burns require hospitalization, but not necessarily at a specialized burn center. A *minor burn* is any partial thickness burn involving less than 15 percent BSA or 10 percent BSA in older adults, and full thickness burns of less than 2 percent BSA that do not involve the face, hands, eyes, ears, feet, or perineum and do not pose any functional or cosmetic risk. Patients with minor burns require transfer to the closest emergency facility, but may not require hospitalization.

Stabilization and Management

Appropriate burn care of elder patients is similar to that of younger adults, and begins with stabilization and treatment in the field and transfer to a burn center or transfer to the closest emergency receiving facility where the patient can be further stabilized prior to subsequent transfer to a burn center.

Stabilization and treatment of elder patients with burns begins with airway, breathing, and circulation. These are the most important functions of the prehospital provider in caring for an elder burn victim. If the patient is the victim of a fire, check for signs of inhalation injury, including dyspnea, mouth or nasal burns, singed nasal hairs, carbonaceous (sooty) sputum, raspy cough, or change in voice. If any of these signs are present, the patient should be placed on humidified, high-flow oxygen via a non-rebreather mask. Elder patients with severe respiratory distress require assisted ventilations and should be intubated as early as possible for airway protection. Patients with severe airway burns can develop sudden airway swelling that can make delayed intubation difficult or impossible. All elder burn victims should also be placed on a cardiac monitor and have a large-bore IV established in a non-burned extremity.

The prehospital provider should always assume that any elder patient exposed to fire and smoke has carbon monoxide poisoning.

This should be assumed even if there is no evidence of airway or skin burns, and even if exposure time was short. Carbon monoxide (CO) is a colorless, odorless, poisonous gas created by incomplete combustion of carbon. Common sources of CO include gas and diesel motors, kerosene heaters, and structural fires. All elder patients with suspected CO poisoning should be removed from the source of CO and placed on high-flow oxygen via a non-rebreather mask. If intubated for respiratory failure or airway burns, elder patients should receive 100 percent oxygen through the endotracheal tube. High-flow oxygen is the best treatment for CO poisoning in the prehospital setting because the high concentration of oxygen increases the removal of CO from hemoglobin in the blood cells. High-flow oxygen should be maintained until the patient has been transferred to the emergency department.

Elder patients with major burns may initially be in shock. If shock is present, elevate the legs immediately and establish a large-bore intravenous line, preferably in an upper extremity but not through burned skin. These patients should be placed on a cardiac monitor. If transport time is expected to be less than 30 min and shock is mild, infusing a lactated ringer's solution or normal saline at a rate of 75 cc/hr should be sufficient. If shock is severe or if transport time is expected to be greater than 30 min and the patient has a burn injury of greater than 20 percent BSA, fluid resuscitation should be initiated. The amount of volume required depends on the patient's clinical status, and should be administered under the direction of the medical control physician.

After initial assessment and stabilization, a complete focused assessment should be performed. Examine the elder patient for fractures and other trauma as well as burns. If possible, obtain information for the medical control physician about underlying medical conditions such as heart disease, emphysema (COPD), and diabetes, which may affect prehospital treatment. Calculate the total BSA burn and categorize the burn into a major, moderate, or minor burn. Burned clothing should be removed, if possible, but without injuring underlying skin. All burned skin should be washed with cool water or saline, and if less than 10 percent of BSA, the burned part can be immersed in cool water or saline, preferably 1–5°C (33.8–41°F), for 30 min. This should be initiated in the field. Immersion therapy has no benefit if delayed more than 30 min after the burn injury, so it should be initiated immediately. Timely immersion therapy results in pain reduction, reduced swelling and intravascular fluid losses, and may limit local vascular insufficiency after burn injury. Smaller burns of less than 9 percent BSA can be immersed longer than 30 min for patient comfort if transport time is prolonged and the patient is stable. Immersion therapy is not indicated in the prehospital setting with larger burns (greater than 10 percent BSA), as there is a risk of hypothermia. Ice should never be applied directly to a burn.

Elder burn victims with extensive burns should be placed on a clean sheet or a sterile burn sheet to prevent contamination and reduce body heat loss. The patient should then be covered with a clean sheet or sterile burn sheet and a clean blanket to minimize heat losses. Under conditions of advanced life support, if transport time is less than 30 min, elder patients with major burns should be transported to a specialized burn center. If transport time is anticipated to be greater than 30 min or if burns are moderate or minor, elder patients can be transferred to the nearest hospital emergency department for further stabilization and treatment. Subsequent transfer to a burn center may be accomplished later, if indicated.

REVIEW QUESTIONS

1. Hypothermia is defined as a temperature of less than _____ °C.
   a. 30
   b. 32
   c. 35
   d. 37

2. All of the following are causes of hypothermia in elders *except*
   a. hypoglycemia
   b. disorders of the thermoregulatory system
   c. hypotension
   d. socioeconomic factors

3. All of the following are symptoms of hypothermia in elders *except*
   a. confusion
   b. fatigue
   c. difficulty walking
   d. poor appetite

4. Which of the following describes moderate hypothermia?
   a. Temperature of 32–35°C, vague symptoms
   b. Temperature of 28–32°C, semiconsciousness, bradycardia
   c. Temperature of less than 28°C, muscular rigidity
   d. Uncontrolled shivering, confusion, slurred speech

5. The "J wave" seen on the monitor or electrocardiogram is seen
   a. on normal tracings
   b. in mild hypothermia
   c. in moderate hypothermia
   d. in severe hypothermia

6. All of the following are true about the prehospital treatment of the severely hypothermic elder patient *except*
   a. if they go into ventricular fibrillation, cardiac defibrillation should be attempted three times
   b. they should be handled with extreme care to avoid ventricular fibrillation

c. intravenous fluids should be prewarmed if possible
d. they should be immediately moved out of the cold environment after initial assessment and C-spine immobilization

7. Heat exhaustion in elders is characterized by all of the following *except*
   a. temperature usually not greater than 39°C (102.2°F)
   b. muscle cramps
   c. diaphoresis
   d. seizures

8. Rapid cooling of the elder patient with suspected heat stroke should begin in the field
   a. because the patient may suddenly go into ventricular fibrillation
   b. because any delay in cooling is associated with a poorer outcome
   c. by immersing the patient in cold water
   d. only if the patient's temperature is 41°C (105.8°F)

9. You arrive at the scene of an elder patient who was burned when he fell into a bathtub of hot water and was unable to get out on his own. He has burns that have blistered on the lower half of his trunk and back, genitals, and both thighs down to the knee. He is in extreme pain. You calculate that he has second degree burns of approximately 30 percent BSA. You classify this burn as a _____ burn when reporting to the medical control physician
   a. minor
   b. moderate
   c. major
   d. lethal

10. The patient described in question 9 should be taken to
    a. the closest hospital emergency department
    b. a regional burn center if transport time is less than 30 min
    c. a regional burn center only if they are in shock
    d. a regional burn center only if they are in cardiac arrest

---

SUGGESTED READING

Rosen, P. and R. Barkin. 1998. *Emergency medicine: Concepts and clinical practice.* New York: Mosby.

11

Psychiatric and Behavioral Emergencies

Rebecca Bollinger Parker, MD, and Brian Wilson, NREMT–P

OBJECTIVES

By the end of this chapter, the prehospital health care provider should be able to:

1 Distinguish between dementia and delirium.
2 Recognize elder depression and suicidal ideation.
3 Recognize substance abuse in elders.
4 Explain categories of elder abuse and neglect.
5 Complete appropriate assessment and stabilization of the elder person with psychiatric and behavioral emergencies.

You respond to a private home for an unknown medical emergency. On arrival, a man tells you that his companion has been "acting strange" for a few days. He states that she has not been eating, sleeping, or bathing. The patient is an elder woman who is sitting at the table, tearing pages out of a magazine. She is dirty and disheveled, and takes no notice of you when you enter the room. When you ask her what the problem is, she states, "You'd have a problem too, if someone was stealing your money and your books. Look at these pictures. The story is all here." When you ask her to elaborate, she just waves her hand at you and continues to tear out pages. Her companion states that she was well but increasingly forgetful until last week. She went to see her physician for abdominal pain. She was given something for "stomach ulcers." He thinks that it was called a Tagamet. She has been taking her medicine regularly. When you go to take her vital signs, she becomes agitated and tells you to go away and leave her alone. With some difficulty, you record a blood pressure of 150/90, a heart rate of 90, and a respiratory rate of 20. Pulse oximetry (Pulse Ox) is 99 percent. You tell her that she must to go to the hospital for more tests. While loading her on the stretcher, she becomes aggressive and hostile. You manage to restrain her, and she shrieks and tries to claw at you all the way to the ambulance. What do you think is the problem with this woman? What additional questions should you ask the patient or her companion? Is she in danger? What additional treatment can you offer her? Are there any medications you should consider giving her? If so, what are the appropriate dosages?

The elder patient with psychiatric and behavioral problems often presents a diagnostic and management challenge to health care providers. Elder patients have different psychiatric presentations than younger patients, and, unfortunately, many health care providers have not been trained to evaluate and treat mental disorders of the elder patient. Because there are few written works to review for reference, we hope this chapter helps prehospital personnel caring for elder patients better understand mental illness, more accurately assess behavioral disorders, and learn more ways to stabilize and treat these patients when they present with psychiatric and behavioral disorders.

ALTERED MENTAL STATUS: DEMENTIA AND DELIRIUM

The elder patient who develops a change in behavior offers a diagnostic challenge to all medical personnel, particularly when the patient has an underlying dementia. Prehospital health care providers are often called to a scene for patients with behavioral changes ranging from violence and aggression to withdrawal and catatonia. The cause of the patients' behavioral change is not always obvious, especially in elders. In elders, the possible causes of these behavioral changes include dementia, a worsening of chronic dementia, or a state known as *delirium.* Next, we discuss dementia and delirium, and then compare the two syndromes in order to distinguish between them.

Dementia

Dementia is a chronic condition that gradually impairs multiple aspects of cognition, especially memory. The elder with dementia develops memory loss and other impairments of speech, motor activities, recognition of objects, planning, and organizing. By definition, these impairments gradually worsen over months and may render a previously functioning member of society unable to function. Nonetheless, people with dementia are alert and attentive without acute fluctuations of mental status. Multiple studies have shown that dementia occurs in 4–6 percent of the elder population.

Alzheimer's disease, the most common cause of dementia, accounts for more than half of all cases. Memory loss is the most common presenting symptom of Alzheimer's disease. Alzheimer's patients may also exhibit changes in personality, fail to perform daily routines, or lose their way in a familiar setting.

The Alzheimer's process is degenerative with a genetic predisposition. When examining the brain tissue of an Alzheimer's patient under a microscope, one sees a pattern of abnormal findings. Although well-trained medical personnel may correctly suspect that a patient has Alzheimer's disease, only a brain biopsy provides a definitive diagnosis. The usual course of Alzheimer's includes death 8–10 years after the onset of memory problems. Alzheimer's disease is irreversible, but some medications may slow the progression of this disease.

Other irreversible causes of dementia include multi-infarct dementia (i.e., multiple small strokes), Parkinson's disease, and other cerebral tissue disorders. Less than 10 percent of the causes of dementia are reversible. The reversible causes include medications, intoxications (e.g., carbon monoxide, heavy metals), nutritional deficits (e.g., thiamine deficiency), and intracranial processes (e.g., tumors, infections, subdural hematomas). The most frequent cause of treatable dementia is major depression.

RETURNING TO THE CASE

The patient is suffering from delirium. She is distracted, cannot focus, and exhibits delusional and paranoid thinking. It may be that she had early dementia prior to this episode, which may further predispose her to delirium. History that may be important includes other medications that she may be taking, fever or signs of infection, excessive vomiting or diarrhea, trauma, alcohol ingestion, suicidal ideation, and medical or psychiatric history. Her companion states that she drinks a bit and has been falling occasionally. He denies knowledge of any serious head injury or loss of consciousness.

Delirium is usually a sign of an underlying medical or pharmacological problem. Approaches to delirium depend on discovering the underlying problem. Your history taking in the home can be essential in making the diagnosis and successfully treating the patient. Delirium can be caused by life-threatening illness such as drug overdose, subdural hematoma, or severe electrolyte abnormalities. In the prehospital setting, your role is to gather as much information as possible and transport the patient safely to the emergency department for further evaluation.

The patient may be very resistant. You must make every effort to protect the patient and yourself. You may need to employ soft restraints and administer small doses of parenteral benzodiazepines (1–2 mg of Ativan® IM or IV) or a phenothiazine (Haldol® 1–5 mg IM or IV) according to local protocols. Always remember that the patient's delirium may be the result of overmedication (*polypharmacy*). Giving additional sedating medications may further compromise the patient's airway or breathing. Always pay attention to the ABCs, even in the face of very distracting behavior on the part of your patient.

Delirium

Delirium is a syndrome of acute alteration in consciousness, attention, and thought processes. Unlike dementia, delirium most often stems from a treatable disease process. Although delirium may occur at any age, this syndrome occurs more frequently in elders. Studies suggest that anywhere from one-tenth to one-half of hospitalized elder medical patients suffer from delirium. Delirium is frequently underdiagnosed, and when delirium is misinterpreted as a sign of mental illness, major medical problems can be overlooked. This can lead to premature death, because delirium carries a high mortality rate, especially when not appropriately treated.

Assessing mental status changes, particularly in the demented patient, can be difficult and can lead to missing the diagnosis of delirium. Of interest, the greatest risk factor for developing delirium is preexisting dementia. Other risk factors include significant coexisting illnesses, older age, medications, trauma (e.g., hip fracture, closed head injury), surgery, and substance abuse.

Clinically, delirium presents as a rapid mental status change over hours to days that waxes and wanes throughout the day. There is a characteristic lack of attention and fluctuating level of alertness, often with worsening at night. The patient may also experience hallucinations (usually visual), delusions, and decreased activity or agitation. The patient's behavior may range from blatant aggression to withdrawal, the latter being more common. Delirious patients show complete cognitive impairment, disorientation, incoherent rambling speech, and may have short-term memory impairment.

Fortunately, delirium is usually the result of a treatable medical disease. The causes of delirium include diseases that alter oxygenation or metabolism of the brain. Many medications subtly alter mental status, and some, particularly anticholinergic medications, can cause delirium. Intoxication or withdrawal from alcohol or sedative hypnotics may also cause delirium. However, elder patients do not suffer from delirium tremens (DTs) because of alcohol withdrawal as often as younger patients.

Vitamin deficiencies, such as Wernicke's syndrome from thiamine deficiency, may cause delirium. In the United States, Wernicke's syndrome is commonly associated with the malnourished alcoholic and presents as mental status changes, altered gait, and changes in ocular movement. Administering glucose before thiamine in those who are thiamine deficient may precipitate Wernicke's syndrome. The most common infectious cause of delirium is urinary tract infections, often asymptomatic in elders. Cardiovascular diseases such as congestive heart failure, cardiac arrhythmia, and myocardial infarction may also present with delirium. There are several neurologic causes of delirium, but acute central nervous system problems are an etiologic factor in less than 10 percent of delirious patients. In rare cases, exacerbations of psychiatric diseases such as schizophrenia or bipolar disorder cause delirium in elders; however, a new onset of these psychiatric diseases rarely occurs in the elder patient. Finally, major depression, discussed later in the chapter, may also cause delirium.

Dementia and Delirium: A Comparison

Distinguishing between dementia and delirium is essential to identify potentially treatable conditions. Unlike dementia, which is chronic and irreversible, delirium most often stems from a reversible disease process, and untreated leads to a high mortality rate. Differentiating between dementia and delirium is difficult because both impair memory and change intellectual capacity. The differences are in the onset of these diseases, the attention span, level of consciousness, fluctuation of mental status, presence of hallucinations, and psychomotor activity of the patient. Delirium represents an acute change with fluctuating degrees of alertness and confusion, whereas the demented patient is generally alert.

Depression

Do not assume that depression is a normal part of aging. Elders frequently do experience age-specific life challenges such as chronic diseases, loss of many loved ones, physical and social isolation, diminished ability to care for themselves, and living on a fixed income. These circumstances may cause a brief reactive depression, but elders should not experience chronic depression as part of the normal aging process.

Depression is less common in elders than in younger cohorts. Statistically, 3–5 percent of older patients are significantly clinically depressed, although 20 percent of elders experience some depressive symptoms. Institutionalized elders demonstrate a higher frequency of depression than other elders. Although elders make fewer attempts at suicide than younger age groups, they are more successful at completing the task.

Overall, the rate of successful suicide increases with age. Although elders make up only 13 percent of the U.S. population, statistics collected by the Center for Disease Prevention and Control between 1980 and 1992 showed that 19 percent of suicides were committed by patients over the age of 65, the highest percentage of all the age cohorts. Elder widowed or divorced men have the highest suicide rate at 2.7 times higher than the rate for elder married men, 1.4 times higher than for never-married elder men, and more than 17 times higher than that for married elder women. Elder men tend to use violent methods such as hanging and guns, whereas women tend to overdose with medication. In general, the following risk factors predispose elders to suicidal behavior: male sex, Caucasian race, disabling and/or painful chronic disease, isolation, family history of depression, recent life changes, history of substance abuse—particularly alcohol, history of suicide attempts, definitive plans for suicide, low income, excess guilt, hopelessness, agitated depression, severe insomnia, and homosexuality.

Diagnostic criteria for depression is the same for all adults. The person must feel depressed or lose interest in favorite activities or both. A depressed person often exhibits weight loss or gain, insomnia or hypersomnia, psychomotor agitation or retardation, fatigue, feelings of worthlessness or guilt, difficulty concentrating, or recurrent thoughts of death. The only difference in depressive symptoms in elders is their tendency to lose weight more frequently, and their reluctance to report suicidal thoughts. Unique clues to suicidal ideation in the elder patient include expressing their wish to join a dead spouse, stating that they will no longer "be here soon," self-devaluing, or giving away all their possessions. Any of these thoughts and actions suggest suicidal intention. Also be aware that although evidence of functional decline in the elder patient may be a sign of dementia or delirium, it also may indicate an underlying major depression. Just as with other adults, if the elder's symptoms follow an event (e.g., the death of a spouse) and last less than 2 weeks, one should consider this a normal grieving response. However, if depressive symptoms last more than 2 weeks, the patient may require treatment for depression.

Depression may be genetic or have any one of several medical causes, including cancers (especially pancreatic), hypothyroidism, strokes, and medications. Unfortunately, many chronic diseases and social stresses can predispose patients to major depression.

It is often difficult to distinguish between dementia and depression. The depressed person may present with cognitive dysfunction. Patients with major depression, however, present with a more acute onset of symptoms and more depressive feelings than those with dementia. Patients with cognitive impairments should be screened for depression.

Major depression in the elder patient is as treatable as depression in the younger patient. Overall, one-third of depressed elders recover with treatment, one-third remain unchanged, and one-third recover and then relapse.

Substance Abuse

In younger patients, alcoholism and drug addiction often become apparent when addictions cause serious occupational, domestic, or legal problems. Comparatively, addiction in elders is uncovered during the work-up of medical or psychiatric complaints. Social isolation helps the elder patient to conceal substance abuse.

The drug elders most commonly abuse is alcohol. The prevalence of alcohol abuse and dependence in the elder population ranges from 0.6 percent to 3.9 percent. In hospitalized elders, this abuse and dependence increases to 8–23 percent. However, the rate of alcohol dependence decreases with age. Although elder men are more likely to be alcoholics, the majority of new-onset elder alcoholics are women. In general, elder alcoholics require more care, have higher morbidity and mortality rates, and decreased functional ability than other elders.

Alcoholism in the elder patient often presents as dyspepsia, insomnia, depression, dementia, or motor vehicle trauma. Always suspect it in the presence of unexplained trauma (e.g., fractures, closed head injury), neurologic problems, nutritional deficiencies (e.g., Wernicke's), liver cirrhosis, or pancreatic disease. Numerous alcoholic patients also suffer from depression and dementia. In fact, many patients are diagnosed with alcoholism while undergoing psychiatric treatment. Many elders do not admit their addiction to alcohol because they fear the social stigma of alcoholism. It is often difficult to diagnose alcoholism in the elder patient because of unusual presentation, underlying memory impairment, and denial by both the elder and family members.

A simple set of questions may help elicit an elder patient's level of addiction. The CAGE questionnaire is a helpful tool in detecting alcoholism. Any patient answering yes to one or more of the CAGE questions may be at risk for alcoholism and requires further questioning (e.g., Did you drink alcohol in the previous 24 hrs or have a current or previous addiction to alcohol?).

The CAGE questionnaire is a screening tool for alcohol dependence. Alcohol dependence is likely if a patient gives 2 or more positive answers to the following questions:

1. Have you ever felt that you should *C*ut down on your drinking?
2. Have people *A*nnoyed you by criticizing your drinking?
3. Have you ever felt *G*uilty about your drinking?
4. Have you ever had a drink first thing in the morning to steady your nerves or get rid of a hangover (*E*ye opener)?

Elders also abuse prescription medications. Sedative hypnotics (e.g., benzodiazepines) are a favorite of older women. Narcotic abuse is less common and generally includes only prescription drugs (e.g., codeine, dilaudid, percocet); nevertheless, elder narcotic addicts share legal, economic, and social problems with their younger counterparts. Although all substance abusers tend to avoid medical care, the elder patient with chronic medical problems and addiction is at great risk for serious consequences—they do not keep appointments, are unable to buy their medications, and lack a stable social network to assist them.

Success rates for drug treatment are independent of age. One Iowa study of drunk drivers found similar recovery rates among elders and younger cohorts. Little is known about recovery rates for other forms of substance abuse in elders.

Elder Abuse

Elder abuse includes physical, emotional, or financial mistreatment. According to current estimations, abuse occurs in 2–5 percent of the elder population. The medical community suspects that only one in six cases of elder abuse is reported. People may avoid reporting incidents of abuse because they cannot identify the problem or are not aware that elder abuse even exists. Abused elders most frequently live with family members. Other abused senior citizens live on their own, and a small minority live in nursing homes. It is critical that the prehospital health care provider consider and recognize elder abuse in all its forms when evaluating the elder patient. A detailed discussion of elder abuse can be found in Chapter 18. Because prehospital providers are the first to evaluate the patient and have the opportunity to see the home environment, they may be the only ones who can recognize abuse and make a life-saving identification and intervention.

Prehospital Behavioral Assessment of Elders

Prehospital health care providers taking a history and performing a physical assessment of elder patients should keep several important points in mind. The health care provider may experience difficulty distinguishing between the normal effects of aging and acute or chronic diseases. The elder patient may have several chronic medical problems simultaneously that give rise to multiple signs and symptoms. Conditions such as poor eye sight, hearing impairment, and patient fatigue usually increase the time spent obtaining an elder's medical history. Not all older patients suffer from hearing loss, so do not assume that you must raise your voice when speaking to them. When taking a history from an elder patient, remember to speak slowly, use terminology they understand, keep eye contact, and give the patient adequate time to answer your questions. To gather a wholly accurate medical picture of the patient, family members or caregivers must often give part or most of the information. Ask specific questions pertaining to medical history and medications, and bring all the patient's medications to the hospital. Do not forget to include medical records from visiting nurses, nursing homes, or physicians.

Obtaining a History

When acquiring a medical history from an elder patient apparently suffering from delirium or dementia, one must interview the elder person as well as family or caregivers. Important questions to ask are: Was the onset of the patient's symptoms rapid or gradual? How exactly has the patient's behavior changed (i.e., what can they not do now that they could do before)? Is the patient's attention span normal or diminished? Is the patient's behavior consistent throughout the day? Does the patient's behavior worsen at night? Does the patient complain of or display any signs of infection, such as cough, fever, diarrhea, or difficulty urinating? Also, assess cardiac and neurologic symptoms. Has the patient had chest pain, shortness of breath, or impaired movement, sensation, speech, or difficulty walking?

If you suspect depression, your history should include questions regarding chronic illnesses, loss of a loved one, changes in living conditions, loss of weight, and social isolation. Do not be afraid to ask straightforward questions when assessing possible suicidal tendencies. If the elder person is suicidal, look for items that might be used to inflict self-harm (e.g., handguns, knives, medications).

A substance abuse history should include what, when, and how much was taken. Has the patient previously suffered from substance abuse? When on the scene, take note of the surroundings. Is there evidence of alcohol or drug ingestion, including beer bottles, pill bottles, or syringes? The CAGE acronym is a helpful tool in suggesting elderly addiction. Forgetfulness, confusion, visual impairment, self-administration of medication, and multiple prescriptions may lead to accidental drug overdose. Always inquire about medications and assess any medication monitoring activity by caregivers.

In cases of possible elder abuse, observe the home environment carefully. Check the condition of the house and the hygiene of the patient. Check the refrigerator for adequate food, and assess the temperature of the home. A poorly ventilated home should prompt suspicions of carbon monoxide poisoning. Watch the patient interact with the caregiver. Does the patient shy away from the caregiver? Look for evidence of unnecessary restraint or lack of bed changing for the bed-ridden patient. When interviewing the caretaker, assess the history for inconsistencies. Passing on information about an elder person's home environment to the emergency department staff can result in a home assessment for safety that may be life saving.

Focused Assessment

There are several important points to consider when conducting the physical examination:

1. The patient may fatigue easily.
2. Elder patients commonly wear many layers of clothing for warmth; this may hamper the examination.
3. Unless it interferes with patient care, one must respect the patient's modesty.
4. Clearly explain all actions before examining a patient.
5. The patient may downplay or deny symptoms to avoid forcible bed rest, hospitalization, or institutionalization.

As with all patients, one must conduct both initial and focused assessment for the elder patient. Determine the patient's level of consciousness. Note whether the patient's current mental status seems chronic or acutely altered. Elder patients often suffer from concurrent illnesses. Pay particular attention to vital signs and respiratory, cardiovascular, and neurological systems. Check for evidence of unexplainable injuries or abuse. Make note of the depressed patient. Examine the patient's skin for evidence of abuse, such as burns and bruising. Check for pressure ulcers, especially on the sacrum and back.

Treatment

Patients suffering from altered mental status require both basic and advanced prehospital care. Basic care includes maintenance of airway and breathing, with nasal or oral airways if necessary, and high-flow oxygen as needed. Patients with a history of COPD require sufficient, but not excessive, concentrations of oxygen to maintain perfusion; follow local protocols. Patients who remain unconscious and unable to protect their own airway may require intubation. Take vital signs, draw blood, and check the blood glucose level. If the patient's blood glucose level is low, this may indicate the need for administration of thiamine and dextrose 50 percent. Consider naloxone (Narcan) if you suspect narcotic overdose. Signs and symptoms include altered mental status, presence of narcotic prescriptions, or pinpoint pupils. Place the patient on the cardiac monitor, as elder patients often have cardiac arrhythmias and underlying cardiac disease. Assess for sufficient cardiac output and treat cardiac compromise according to local protocols.

Restraining the patient is appropriate in certain circumstances. Remember that delirium requiring restraint is often a symptom of an underlying medical problem. Also, remember delirious patients do not act deliberately when belligerent or combative. Unnecessary aggression or force with elder patients will predictably worsen the situation. Although restraining methods and guidelines are similar for all patients, elders are more prone to injury from excessive or insufficient restraint. Restraints should hold the patient securely without compromising circulatory or respiratory status. Soft restraints should be used whenever possible. Stretcher straps can also be used to restrain an agitated patient, but the chest strap should be loosely applied. Remember to assess distal pulses after the application of restraints. Remember that underlying medical conditions may hinder placing the patient in a prone position, so the patient may need to be placed in another position while restrained. A continuing evaluation of vital signs and careful monitoring is essential for patient safety. In the depressed uncooperative patient with suicidal ideation, keep in mind that the prehospital health care provider often must transport the patient against his or her will. Follow local laws and protocols and contact the medical control physician for guidance.

Treatment for physical abuse depends on the type of injuries sustained. Physical abuse is the least common of the four types of elder abuse, and signs and symptoms vary. Treat traumatic injuries as indicated. Most states require mandatory reporting of elder abuse by law. All states have adult protective services or similar state agencies that help possible elder abuse victims. These agencies assess the living environment and offer legal assistance if necessary. A more extensive discussion of this topic can be found in Chapter 18. Refer to your local jurisdiction for further details. Always remember that the mentally competent patient may refuse transport. Carefully counsel the patient about the risks of staying in an abusive and potentially life-threatening environment. In most states, reporting requirements still apply, even if the patient refuses transport.

CASE OUTCOME

To transport the patient safely, you must use soft restraints. Haloperidal (Haldol®) 5 mg IV was given in the emergency department to calm and sedate the patient for evaluation. In the emergency department, the patient had a negative CT scan of the head, normal blood chemistries, a negative toxicology screen, and a normal lumbar puncture. The physician concludes that Tagamet induced her delirium. The medication is withdrawn and she quickly improves. She is discharged on the third hospital day. Social services counsels her about her alcohol intake and arranges for a home helper.

CONCLUSIONS

1. Changes in mental status in elders often have an underlying medical cause.

2. A complete assessment demands discussion with a caregiver.

3. Dementia makes assessment of mental status changes even more difficult. Try to determine the patient's baseline status and any change.

4. Depression is common. Always evaluate for suicide risk.

5. Prehospital health care providers have an opportunity and obligation to discover abuse and prevent further abuse by assessing the home environment and caretaker relationship. These observations should be conveyed to the emergency department staff.

REVIEW QUESTIONS

1. Which of the following is true about dementia in elders?
   a. Patient's confusion may change throughout the day.
   b. It usually begins suddenly.
   c. Some forms of dementia are reversible.
   d. Dementia occurs in more than 50 percent of the elder population.

2. All of the following are risk factors for delirium *except*
   a. significant coexisting illness
   b. trauma
   c. elder abuse
   d. medications

3. One of the main differences between delirium and dementia is that delirium
   a. usually has a treatable underlying medical cause
   b. is usually not reversible
   c. has a gradual onset over months to years
   d. is only a result of medication side effects

4. All are true about the clinical presentation of delirium *except*
   a. It is a rapid mental status change that may occur over several hours.
   b. There are usually fluctuations in the level of mental alertness, especially at night.
   c. Hallucinations and agitation may occur.
   d. Elder patients with delirium are always alert mentally.

5. Depression in elder patients
   a. occurs most often in institutionalized patients
   b. is more common than in younger patients
   c. rarely results in suicide
   d. is a natural process of aging

6. All are risk factors for suicide in the elder patient *except*
   a. painful or disabling chronic disease
   b. isolation
   c. female sex
   d. substance abuse

7. The most commonly abused drug in the elder population is
   a. alcohol
   b. sedatives
   c. narcotics
   d. amphetamines

8. Alcoholism is common in elder patients with all of the following problems *except*
   a. motor vehicle accident trauma
   b. depression

c. pancreatic disease

d. delirium

9. You respond to the home of an 80-year-old man who is too weak to get out of bed. He appears frail, but his vital signs are stable. He says little, but he is not confused. He has several bruises on his forearms. His daughter-in-law is his caretaker and she does not allow him to answer your questions—she answers them herself. The patient does not make eye contact with his daughter-in-law. You suspect

a. depression

b. dementia

c. elder abuse

d. dehydration

10. All of the following are true about properly treating and transporting a combative elder patient *except*

a. using force to restrain an elder patient may make their agitation worse

b. using IV sedation is almost always necessary

c. distal pulses should be checked after the application of restraints

d. elders are more prone to injury from excessively tight or loose restraints

SUGGESTED READING

American Psychiatric Association. 1994. *Diagnostic and statistical manual of mental disorders: DSM–IV,* 4th ed. Washington D.C.: American Psychiatric Press.

Folstein, M. F. 1997. Geriatric psychiatry: What's new about the old. *The Psychiatric Clinics of North America* 20(1):45–57.

Hazzard, W. R., E. L. Bierman, J. P. Blass, W. H. Ettinger, and J. B. Halter, eds. 1994. *Principles of geriatric medicine and gerontology,* 3d ed. New Baskerville: McGraw-Hill.

Rosen, P. ed. 1992. *Emergency Medicine: Concepts and Clinical Practice,* 3d ed. St. Louis: Mosby–Year Book.

Rubin, E. H. 1997. Geriatric psychiatry: What's new about the old. *The Psychiatric Clinics of North America* 20(1):77–89.

Saunders, A. B. ed. 1996. *Emergency care of the elder person.* St. Louis: Beverly Cracom Publications.

Wooley, D. C. 1997. Geriatric psychiatry: What's new about the old. *The Psychiatric Clinics of North America* 20(1):241–260.

SECTION III

Trauma

12

Head/Spinal Trauma

Liudvikas Jagminas, MD

OBJECTIVES

By the end of this chapter, the prehospital health care provider should be able to:

1 List the common causes of head and spinal injury in elders.

2 Define the signs and symptoms of the following conditions:
Skull fracture
Intracranial injury
Increased intracranial pressure
Cushing's triad
Cervical spine injury
Neurogenic shock
Spinal shock

3 Perform a careful initial assessment when central nervous system (CNS) trauma is present.

4 Identify the proper care steps for the following conditions:
Head injury with decreased level of consciousness
Cervical spine injury

CASE

You are called to a local shopping mall for a woman who has fallen down several stairs. On arrival, you find an elder woman lying at the bottom of the stairs, awake but confused. A bystander states that there was no loss of consciousness. On physical examination, she has a blood pressure of 200/110, a heart rate of 60, a respiratory rate of 26, and a pulse oximetry reading of 99 percent on room air. She has a large contusion on her forehead. Her pupils are equal, round, and reactive to light. She has mild neck tenderness without deformity. Her lungs are clear, and her abdomen is soft. Although she has no deformities or tenderness of her extremities, you note that her upper extremities are weak, but her lower extremity strength seems normal. What do you think is the problem with this woman? What additional history should be obtained? What prehospital stabilization and treatment should you initiate prior to hospital transfer?

The general management principles for elder patients with head and neck trauma are similar to the general population, but there are important differences in the etiology and outcome of head and neck trauma. Head trauma is the leading cause of death in all trauma patients. Victims of head trauma most frequently are young adult males involved in motor vehicle accidents. However, morbidity, mortality and prolonged neuropsychiatric deficits are much higher in the elderly. Patients older than 65 years of age with a Glasgow Coma Scale (GCS) of 8 or less have a mortality of about 90 percent. This is second only to shock as a predictor of overall mortality. *Minor head trauma,* defined as a GCS of 13–15 and only a brief loss of consciousness, can be devastating in elders. Mortality in elders after minor head trauma is 5 percent, compared with only 0.35 percent in younger patients. In addition, elder patients who survive head trauma are hospitalized longer and are left with greater neurologic deficits. The reasons for poorer outcomes are the possibility of pre-existing brain injury and underlying brain disease including hydrocephalus (an increased amount of fluid within the cranial cavity), Alzheimer's disease, and microvascular (small blood vessel) disease. In addition, elders frequently suffer from other medical conditions, such as cardiovascular disease (resulting in hypoperfusion of brain tissue) and pulmonary disease (resulting in hypoxia), and they often take blood thinners that can worsen head injury by causing increased bleeding.

Falls are the most common cause of injury in elders, followed by pedestrian accidents. The age of the patient appears to influence the type of brain injury seen. Epidural hematomas are almost nonexistent in elders, whereas subdural hematomas are three times more likely. One likely reason for the scarcity of epidural hematomas in this age range is because as the brain ages, the dura (the tough tissue covering the brain) adheres more tightly to the skull. There are multiple reasons for the increased likelihood of subdural hematomas. These include increased fragility of veins, cerebral atrophy (leading to increased stretching of the bridging veins), and a greater tendency to bleed from either medications or illness. The cerebral atrophy associated with aging allows an intracranial hematoma to expand more easily, and allows gradual development of symptoms. Generally, there are no signs or symptoms to distinguish a subdural hematoma from a cerebral contusion. The diagnosis of a subdural hematoma should be considered in any elder patient complaining of a headache, with mental status changes or exhibiting gait disturbances, whether or not neurologic deficits are present. Remember that a history of head trauma is lacking in up to 50 percent of elder patients who are ultimately diagnosed with subdural hematomas. Even minor head trauma can have a poor or even fatal outcome. In one study, 20 percent of elder patients evaluated for head trauma who had a GCS of 13 or greater had massive hematomas, and 12 percent expired.

Brain injury as a result of trauma can be divided into primary and secondary etiologies. *Primary brain injury* occurs on impact, and brain tissue undergoes varying degrees of injury to the neurons and axons that make up the brain cells. These injuries to the brain cells currently cannot be treated. *Secondary brain injury* occurs from potentially treatable factors such as intracranial hemorrhage, cerebral edema, ischemia, and increased intracranial pressure. In addition, easily preventable factors, such as hypoxia, hypercarbia, and hypertension, play a major role in morbidity and mortality. Optimal management of the elder head injured patient requires attention to such treatable factors to minimize secondary brain injury and improve neurologic recovery.

INTRACRANIAL PRESSURE

The contents of the skull, including cerebrospinal fluid, blood, blood vessels, and brain matter, are relatively noncompressible. If there is an increase in volume in any one of these components it must be offset by an equal decrease in one of the other components or intracranial pressure (ICP) rises.

The brain has autoregulation that helps maintain normal ICP (<15 mmHg) in the face of an increasing mass. However, once those compensatory mechanisms can no longer accommodate the expanding mass, the ICP begins to rise dramatically. Once the ICP rises to the level of systemic arterial pressure (SAP), cerebral perfusion stops and brain death results.

Herniation

Uncontrolled increased ICP can result in transtentorial or uncal herniation. In this situation, the increase in pressure in the skull starts to push the brain tissue against fixed structures in the skull, causing abnormal brain function. This results in two findings, a mid-fixed pupil on the same side as the compressive lesion with paralysis opposite to the side of the abnormal pupil. Continued brain stem compression results in deterioration in the level of consciousness leading to coma, hyperventilation, bradycardia, and hypertension (Cushing's triad).

Cerebral Concussion

Cerebral concussion is a traumatic and temporary loss of consciousness with possible associated memory loss but without underlying structural brain injury. These injuries are generally associated with minor transient neurologic deficits and cause no permanent brain damage.

Cerebral Contusion

Cerebral contusion occurs when severe acceleration and deceleration forces are applied to the head and cause the brain to impact on sharp bony outcroppings within the cranium. Neurologic deficits vary depending on the site of brain injury. Generally, there is a loss of consciousness, lasting from several minutes up to 1 hr or more. *Anterograde* (after the event) or *retrograde* (before the event) amnesia and vomiting may be present. Cerebral contusion can occur in the same area as the head injury, or can occur in an area opposite to the head injury (contracoup injury).

Cerebral Laceration

A cerebral laceration is a severe injury of the brain matter with more severe and lasting neurologic deficits than cerebral concussion or contusion.

Skull Fracture

Because of the round shape of the skull, a large amount of force is required to cause a fracture. Eighty percent of fractures are linear, and the remainder are depressed, open, comminuted (crushed), or basilar in nature.

It is difficult, at best, to detect a skull fracture by physical examination, but the prehospital health care provider should suspect such a fracture if the mechanism of injury is suggestive. Basilar skull fractures can be diagnosed by physical examination. Raccoon eyes (dark bruising around the eyes) are indicative of frontal basilar skull fractures, whereas Battle's sign (dark bruising behind the ear at the base of the skull) is indicative of an occipital skull fracture. The prehospital health care provider should keep in mind that these two findings take several hours to develop, and may not be evident at the scene.

RETURNING TO THE CASE

This patient has a head injury and is at significant risk for a spinal cord injury. As you secure her airway and immobilize her cervical spine, she tells you that she takes a "blood thinner" and "a pill" for her diabetes. She is unable to name her medications. The cardiac monitor shows atrial fibrillation with a ventricular rate of 62. Her arms are so weak that she cannot place them across her chest when asked to do so. You carefully secure her to the backboard, cover her with warm blankets, and prepare to transfer her to the hospital. A blood sugar checked en route to the hospital is normal.

Intracranial Hematomas

Field diagnosis of intracranial hematomas is difficult. Understanding the essential features of intracranial hematomas ensures that the prehospital health care provider can report pertinent information to medical control and that the patient is transported to the appropriate facility.

Epidural hematoma. Epidural hematoma results from arterial bleeding between the dura mater and the inner table of the skull. They represent about 2 percent of head injuries requiring hospitalization. Approximately 20 percent of all patients with epidural hematoma die even if properly diagnosed and treated. As mentioned earlier, epidural hematomas are almost nonexistent in elders.

In general, these injuries are the result of low-velocity blows to the head, and are often associated with a skull fracture that lacerates the middle meningeal artery. After an initial period of unconsciousness, there is an intervening "lucid period," during which the patient seems normal, lasting minutes to several hours before there is a lapse back into unconsciousness. Upwards of 20 percent of patients never exhibit the "lucid period." This injury necessitates rapid stabilization and transport for neurosurgical intervention.

Subdural hematoma. Subdural hematomas generally occur as the result of venous bleeding between the dura mater and the brain.

Frequently there is an associated underlying brain injury. This type of injury is three times more frequent in elders than in the general population because the intracranial veins become more fragile and stretched because of cerebral atrophy associated with aging. In addition, elder patients are more likely to be on anticoagulants or suffer from blood clotting deficiencies. Subdural hematomas have been termed the *great imitator* because the presenting signs and symptoms vary greatly. A patient may have an early loss of consciousness and focal motor signs immediately after trauma, or may only complain of a mild headache, subtle mental status changes, or a new gait disturbance. In elder patients with subdural hematoma, a history of trauma is frequently lacking.

Intracerebral hematoma. These injuries can occur with penetrating head injury or with sudden and severe accelerating and decelerating injury. This leads to a laceration or tearing of blood vessels within brain tissue. Seizure activity is a common sign with this type of injury. Focal neurologic signs and symptoms depend on the area of injured brain tissue.

SPINAL INJURY

Cervical spine injury is present from 6 percent to 60 percent of patients with head or facial trauma. Injury to the cervical spine may present with minimal neurologic complaints such as weakness, numbness, or tingling of the extremities. The prehospital health care provider must always remember that the signs and symptoms of serious cervical spine injury in the elder patient may be subtle. Any seemingly minor mechanism, physical complaint, or finding may represent a catastrophic underlying cervical spine injury.

Elders are at risk for spinal injury for several age-related reasons:

1. Chronic bony changes with stiffening of the spine.
2. Bony spur formation with impingement into the spinal canal.
3. Osteoporosis.

All of these changes place the spine of the elder patient at increased risk for fracture, and the spinal cord at risk for damage following even minor trauma. An increased level of suspicion with strict adherence to spinal immobilization on the part of the prehospital health care provider is required to prevent further injury and to preserve neurologic outcome.

Detection of spinal injuries in elders may be quite difficult. History taking and clinical evaluation may be unreliable in some patients because of Alzheimer's dementia or other underlying neurologic impairment. Arthritic and degenerative changes contribute to making the examination difficult because it may not be possible to differentiate preexisting chronic neck pain from that as a result of acute injury.

It has been estimated that 13,000 new spinal cord injuries occur every year. Motor vehicle accidents and falls account for 54 percent of new spinal cord injuries. The remainder are the result of firearms and recreational activities.

After a survey of the scene and the mechanism of injury, the prehospital health care provider should immediately control and immobilize the head and neck of the patient. Next a semirigid collar and spinal immobilization board should be applied and secured. No collar can adequately immobilize the occiput, C1 and C2. This can only be accomplished by securing the head to the spinal board with pads and straps or tape and sandbags. All patients with posttraumatic spinal pain or tenderness, unconsciousness, intoxication because of drugs or alcohol, neurologic findings (such as a weak extremities), parasthesias (tingling) of the extremities, a distracting painful injury or a suspicious mechanism of injury must have their cervical spine fully and securely immobilized.

SPINAL CORD SYNDROMES

Spinal cord syndromes can be categorized into two types: incomplete and complete. Of the incomplete traumatic cord syndromes, *central cord syndrome* is by far the most common in elders. It usually results from a hyperextension neck injury (this occurs when the head is forced backward) in persons with a narrow spinal canal as a result of spondylosis (degenerative changes of the vertebrae associated with aging). Generally, the patient has weakness that is worse in the arms than in the legs. The weakness is also worse in the hands than in the muscles of the upper arms. Urinary retention is common with a variable sensory deficit below the level of the cord injury. It is important to differentiate this syndrome from a complete cord injury because the prognosis is dramatically different.

Complete spinal cord injury results from a complete transection of the spinal cord. The result is that all cord function is absent below the level of injury. Recovery of any neurologic function below that level is generally minimal.

Neurogenic shock refers to blood pressure instability because of loss of vascular tone. These patients typically have a systolic blood pressure of 80–100 mmHg yet have warm, dry skin, and either normal heart rates or bradycardia. Priapism (penile erection) may serve as a sign of spinal cord injury, along with loss of bowel control and urinary retention.

Severe injury to the spinal cord may cause *spinal shock,* which differs from neurogenic shock. Spinal shock leads to sudden, transient loss of reflexes in the distal extremities, which can last hours to weeks. The patient initially presents with a flaccid quadriplegia (no muscle tone in the arms or legs). As spinal shock resolves (usually within 24 hr) reflexes return, and the patient develops a spastic paralysis.

ASSESSMENT

Because the elder head-injured patient may be unconscious or have a diminished level of consciousness, it may be impossible to get an accurate history of the events leading up to the injury. Talking with bystanders and surveying the scene to get a sense of the forces involved in the injury is important. If the patient was involved in a motor vehicle crash, look for clues of body contact such as a starred windshield, bent steering wheel, or broken dashboard. These clues can yield information about how forces were transmitted to the body.

The assessment of the elder trauma patient basically follows the same guidelines as those applied to any adult patient. The prehospital health care provider must make an initial assessment of the airway, breathing, and circulation (ABCs) with attention to cervical spine immobilization, followed by the focused assessment. Special attention should be paid to the following areas:

Large-bore IVs, cardiac monitoring, and supplemental oxygen, with frequent vital sign monitoring.

History taking and clinical examination may be difficult or even unreliable as a result of underlying neurologic problems, Alzheimer's, dementia, or impaired hearing.

Arthritic and degenerative changes and preexisting conditions may make the examination difficult and it may not be possible to differentiate acute injury from a chronic syndrome.

Severe arthritic conditions, especially in the cervical region may prevent patient from being immobilized in the usual fashion.

Elders are more likely to have dentures or other material in the mouth that must be removed to facilitate a protected airway.

Oxygen supplementation is important because of increased incidence of cardiovascular disease.

Thermal protection must be maintained because elders are prone to heat loss because of decreased fat reserves.

All head-injured patients should be suspected of having a cervical spine injury and be managed accordingly.

Airway: Rapid assessment and maintenance of a patent airway is vital, but may be difficult to achieve because of the need for

C-spine precautions and the presence or absence of dentures. Jaw thrust or chin lift maneuvers should be employed in these cases.

Breathing: Head injury may produce several types of abnormal respiratory patterns. As ICP rises, the respiratory rate initially slows, then rises as ICP continues to rise, then slows and ultimately stops if the rising ICP is not corrected.

Blood Pressure: Severe head injury with elevated ICP will cause an increase in the systolic blood pressure with ultimate widening of the pulse pressure.

Hypotension as the result of an isolated closed head injury is rare and if present it is usually a terminal event. If a patient with a head injury is hypotensive, other causes of hypotension must be explored. Note the pulse rate. Bradycardia may be related to an elevated ICP when associated with hypertension and an irregular respiratory pattern (Cushing's triad).

Control the cervical spine: Use a rigid collar, backboard, and tape.

Disability: Make a rapid assessment of the level of consciousness, level of orientation, and response to stimuli using the acronym AVPU; Awake, Verbal stimuli to arouse, Painful stimuli to arouse, and Unresponsive. Assess the GCS and any weakness or inability to move extremities, as well as pupillary size and response. Carefully monitor the neurologic status for any deterioration.

Neurologic Examination

During the initial assessment, the level of consciousness should be assessed by the acronym AVPU. Pupilary size and response should be noted along with motor and sensory examination.

Head and Spinal Examination

The head should be visually inspected for signs of trauma, impaled objects, bleeding, deformity or fluid leaking from the ears or nose. Palpation should include the scalp for any open wounds or impaled objects, the face for instability or crepitus (a crunching or crackling under the skin with palpation) and the neck for point tenderness or expanding hematomas. Any patient with the following should be properly immobilized:

Trauma of the clavicles or above.
Mechanism of injury suggestive of head or neck injury.
History of loss of consciousness.
Alteration of consciousness.
Obvious neurologic deficit.
Drug or alcohol intoxication.

The patient is taken to a nearby trauma center. She is evaluated by the emergency physician as well as a trauma specialist. A CT scan of her head shows a large right subdural hematoma. During her emergency department evaluation, her mental status deteriorates and she is intubated with careful in-line stabilization of the cervical spine. A plain x-ray of the cervical spine shows a possible fracture of the 5th cervical vertebra and possible hyperextension injury. She is given clotting factors to reverse the warfarin (Coumadin®) she is taking and is given steroids for her presumed spinal cord injury. She is taken to the operating room for removal of her subdural hematoma. Following surgery, she has a magnetic resonance imaging (MRI) scan showing a central cord syndrome. She later has surgery to stabilize her cervical fracture, and after 2 weeks is transferred to a rehabilitation hospital. There she recovers enough function to live independently at home.

MANAGEMENT

The prehospital management of an elder patient with suspected head or neck trauma should focus on the prevention of secondary injury, the maintenance of cervical spine stability and cerebral perfusion pressure. This can be accomplished by spinal immobilization, providing high-flow oxygen and preventing hypercarbia (high levels of CO_2 in the bloodstream) and hypotension.

As with any patient, the ABCs are paramount. In an attempt to secure or maintain an airway, endotracheal intubation with in-line immobilization may be required. After a head injury, vomiting is often a problem. Therefore, aggressive airway protection to prevent aspiration, aggressive suctioning, and having the patient secured to the backboard in case they need to be rolled to one side is vital.

REVIEW QUESTIONS

1. Mortality in elders after head trauma is about
   a. 5 percent
   b. 10 percent
   c. 25 percent
   d. 50 percent

2. All are reasons that elders have poorer outcomes after head trauma *except*
   a. blood thinners
   b. cardiovascular disease

c. diabetes

d. Alzheimer's disease

3. Subdural hematomas in the elder population
    a. occur only if the patient is taking warfarin (Coumadin®)
    b. may be present even if there is no history of head injury
    c. are less common than epidural hematomas
    d. are caused only by major head trauma

4. All of the following are potentially treatable causes of secondary brain injury *except*
    a. intracranial hemorrhage
    b. brain edema
    c. brain ischemia
    d. direct injury to neurons and axons during head trauma

5. The major difference between cerebral concussion and cerebral contusion is
    a. cerebral concussion usually results in permanent neurologic deficits
    b. cerebral contusion is more severe and results from the brain hitting bony outcroppings in the cranium
    c. cerebral concussion often causes amnesia and vomiting
    d. cerebral contusion usually results in only transient neurologic deficits

6. All of the following are reasons that elders are predisposed to spinal injury *except*
    a. weakening of the muscles of the neck
    b. osteoporosis
    c. stiffening of the spine
    d. bony spur formation with impingement into the spinal canal

7. The prehospital health care provider plays a critical role in the care of the elder patient with suspected cervical spine injury
    a. by recognizing that even minor head or neck injury can result in a cervical spine fracture
    b. by immobilizing the cervical spine to prevent additional neurologic injury
    c. by immobilizing the cervical spine to preserve neurologic outcome
    d. all of the above

8. All of the following are characteristic of a central cord syndrome in an elder patient *except*
    a. it usually occurs as a result of hyperextension of the neck
    b. weakness is greater in the arms than in the legs
    c. urinary retention frequently occurs
    d. complete paralysis below the level of the injury

9. You are at the scene of a motor vehicle crash involving an elder man with a major head injury. He is unconscious and hypotensive. You suspect
    a. intracranial hemorrhage
    b. subdural hematoma

    c. Cushing's triad

    d. another injury may be causing the hypotenison

10. All of the following elder patients with suspected C-spine injury should be immobilized *except*

    a. those intoxicated by drugs or alcohol

    b. those with injuries to the clavicles or above

    c. those with loss of consciousness

    d. all of the above

SUGGESTED READING

Amacher, A. L. and D. E. Bybee. 1987. Toleration of head injury by the elderly. *Neurosurgery* 20(6):954–958.

Biffl, W. L., F. A. Moore, E. E. Moore, A. Sauaia, R. A. Read, and J. M. Burch. 1994. Cardiac enzymes are irrelevant in the patient with suspected myocardial contusion. *American Journal of Surgery* 168(6):523–527.

Choi, S. C., T. Y. Barnes, R. Bullock, T. A. Germanson, A. Marmarous, and H. F. Young. 1994. Temporal profile of outcomes in severe head injury. *Journal of Neurosurgery* 81(2):169–173.

DeMaria, E. J., P. R. Kenney, M. A. Merriam, L. A. Casanova, and D. S. Gann. 1987. Survival after trauma in geriatric patients. *Annals of Surgery* 206(6):738–743.

Gennarelli, T. A., H. R. Champion, W. J. Sacco, W. S. Copes, and W. M. Alves. 1989. Mortality of patients with head injury and extracranial injury treated in trauma centers. *Journal of Trauma* 29(9):1193–1202.

Jackimczyk, K. 1993. Blunt chest trauma. *Emergency Medical Clinics of North America* 11(1):81–96.

Lonner, J. H. and K. J. Koval. 1995. Polytrauma in the elderly. *Clinical Orthopedics and Related Research* (318):136–143.

Nelson, R. C. and M. A. Amin. 1990. Falls in the elderly. *Emergency Medical Clinics of North America* 8(2):309–324.

Pellicane, J. V., K. Byrne, and E. J. DeMaria. 1992. Preventable complications and death from multiple organ failure among geriatric trauma victims. *Journal of Trauma* 33(3):440–444.

Saywell Jr., R. M., J. R. Woods, S. A. Rappaport, and T. L. Allen. 1989. The value of age and severity as predictors of costs in geriatric head trauma patients. *Journal of the American Geriatric Society* 37(7):625–630.

Shackford, S. R., S. L. Wald, S. E. Ross, T. H. Cogbill, D. B. Hoyt, J. A. Morris, P. A. Mucha, H. L. Pachter, H. J. Sugerman, K. O'Malley, et al. 1992. The clinical utility of computed tomographic scanning and neurologic examination in the management of patients with minor head injuries. *Journal of Trauma* 33(3):385–394.

van Aalst, J. A., J. A. Morris Jr., H. K. Yates, R. S. Miller, and S. M. Bass. 1991. Severely injured geriatric patients return to independent living: A study of factors influencing function and independence. *Journal of Trauma* 31(8):1096–1101.

van der Sluis, C. K., H. J. Klasen, W. H. Eisma, and H. J. ten Duis. 1996. Major trauma in young and old: What is the difference? *Journal of Trauma* 40(1):78–82.

Weiss, R. L., J. A. Brier, W. O'Connor, S. Ross, and C. M. Brathwaite. 1996. The usefulness of transesophageal echocardiography in diagnosing cardiac contusions. *Chest* 109(1):73–77.

Wilberger, J. E., Jr., M. Harris, and D. L. Diamond. 1991. Acute subdural hematoma: Morbidity, mortality, and operative timing. *Journal of Neurosurgery* 74(2):212–218.

Woolard, R. H., B. M. Becker, and T. Haronian. 1995. Geriatric considerations. In *The clinical practice of emergency medicine,* ed. A. Harwood-Nuss 1559–1565. Philadelphia: Lippincott.

Zietlow, S. P., P. J. Capizzi, M. P. Bannon, and M. B. Farnell. 1994. Multisystem geriatric trauma. *Journal of Trauma* 37(6):985–988.

13

Chest Trauma

Alex Lee, MD

OBJECTIVES

By the end of this chapter, the prehospital health care provider should be able to:

1 Classify the types of chest injures.

2 Recognize and treat chest injuries in elders that require immediate attention.

3 Describe signs and symptoms associated with each chest injury.

4 Discuss the assessment and treatment of chest trauma in elder patients.

You respond to the home of a elder man who has fallen 10 feet from a ladder onto his cement driveway. He has had no loss of consciousness and complains only of pain on the left side of his chest where he hit the ground. He denies any prior medical problems and takes no medications. On examination he is alert and oriented and in mild respiratory distress. His vital signs are blood pressure 120/70, heart rate 110, and respiratory rate 32. He is able to take only shallow respirations because of pain, and his lung sounds are diminished on the left. He has a large abrasion and contusion on his left chest wall and has several obvious rib fractures. He has minor abrasions of his upper and lower extremities and no other apparent injuries. You provide supplemental oxygen, place him on the cardiac monitor, and immobilize his cervical spine with a rigid collar and backboard. You establish an IV with normal saline running at a maintenance rate. As you prepare to place him in the ambulance, he becomes more tachypneic and tachycardic. You are unable to hear any breath sounds on the left. What do you think is the problem with this man? Is he in danger? What prehospital stabilization and treatment should you initiate prior to hospital transfer?

One of the most frequently encountered prehospital emergency medical problems of elder patients is a history of trauma. Studies demonstrate that injured elder persons differ from their young counterparts in the cause of their injuries, their response to injuries, and their outcome. Just as children are not just small adults, health care professionals are beginning to appreciate that elder persons are not just old adults.

ETIOLOGY

Chest trauma is second only to head injury as a leading cause of traumatic death and accounts for approximately one of every four trauma deaths in this country. Despite these facts, fewer than 15 percent of all chest injuries treated require operative intervention. The remaining injuries require only relatively basic supportive therapy and observation, started as soon as possible after the onset of injury. Improved emergency services and rapid transport of injured patients has increased the number of elder survivors of chest injuries. Many of these patients would once have died at the scene or in transit. Prehospital health care providers must understand the pathophysiology of chest trauma in elders and be prepared to intervene in these critically injured patients.

Table 13.1.   Thoracic Injuries Requiring Immediate Intervention

Flail chest
Pneumothorax (tension, open)
Massive hemothorax
Cardiac tamponade
Traumatic asphyxia

This chapter reviews the assessment, stabilization, and treatment of chest injuries involving the cardiopulmonary system. First, we discuss thoracic injuries that require immediate intervention (Table 13.1), followed by thoracic injuries that require monitoring and stabilization (Table 13.2).

Chest injuries can be the result of either blunt or penetrating trauma. Penetrating injuries are usually obvious and usually involve either a gunshot or knife wound. Blunt trauma is a greater diagnostic difficulty, as major life-threatening injuries may not be obvious on initial examination. There can be significant damage to the chest wall, heart, great vessels, lungs, trachea, esophagus, and diaphragm. Many of these injuries are difficult to diagnose even in the hospital setting. The goal is to gather as much information as possible in the limited time available to identify any potential injury that may be present. This suspicion may result in a difference in therapy or triage designation that may be important to the patient's chance of recovery.

Several conditions that can benefit from immediate prehospital intervention are flail chest, pneumothorax, massive hemothorax, tension pneumothorax, cardiac tamponade, and traumatic asphyxia.

Flail Chest

Flail chest is a result of blunt trauma, and can occur when a patient's chest impacts the steering wheel in a motor vehicle crash, or as a

Table 13.2.   Thoracic Injuries Requiring Monitoring and Stabilization

Simple rib fracture
Clavicular fracture
Sternal fracture
Pulmonary contusion
Myocardial contusion
Tracheobronchial injuries
Aorta and great vessel injury
Diaphragmatic and esophageal injury

result of a fall. Usually three or more ribs are fractured in two or more places each, making the chest unstable. The sternum or the cartilaginous attachments to the chest may also be involved. *Kyphosis* (bending of the spinal column) is present in two-thirds of elder patients and chest wall elasticity is reduced, resulting in less chest wall compliance, and a greater risk of rib or sternal fractures. Because the chest wall is more rigid in elder patients, they are more likely to have multiple rib fractures after blunt chest trauma. Paradoxical respirations result with the flail segment moving as a result of intrathoracic pressures rather than muscular control. The side of the chest with fractures is pulled in during inhalation, preventing complete expansion of the lung, and pushed outward during exhalation. The paradox is that this movement is the opposite of what normally happens during respiration. Under this circumstance, the lung fails to ventilate properly and the patient oxygenates poorly, although respiratory effort may appear adequate. The prehospital health care provider must keep in mind that in the elder patient, this flail segment is often not apparent because of either shallow respirations or muscle splinting. The high morbidity associated with a flail chest injury is not from the sometimes dramatic movement of the chest, but instead from the patient's reluctance to take a deep breath and cough. This frequently leads to hypoventilation, collapse of the airways, and pneumonia.

Observation of the chest for paradoxical movements is the most important point in the recognition of a flail chest. A high index of suspicion may also be needed if the patient is muscular because as pain can cause muscular splinting, it may be difficult to see the flail movement. Although painful to the patient, palpation of the chest may reveal crepitus and possibly the disconnected rib section. Age over 65 is an indication for early ventilatory support with a bag–valve mask or endotracheal intubation in patients with flail chest, as mortality is significantly higher in elderly patients who are intubated only after the onset of respiratory failure.

Pneumothorax

A pneumothorax occurs when an internal or external injury allows air, blood, or fluid to enter the pleural cavity. Expansion of the pleural space reduces the effective lung expansion and compromises respirations. If the pleural cavity expands because of an alveolar (internal) injury, it is called a *closed pneumothorax.* Many elder patients have underlying lung disease, such as emphysema. Weak alveolar tissue can rupture even after minimal chest trauma and cause a pneumothorax. If the wound is external and exposed to the atmosphere, it is called an *open pneumothorax.* Penetrating open chest wounds occur when an object tears or punctures the chest wall, opening the thoracic cavity to the atmosphere. The object may be impaled in the chest wall.

Tension Pneumothorax

A tension pneumothorax can be life threatening. It occurs when there is a tear of the lung, allowing air to escape to the area between the lung and the chest wall. This pleural space is called a *potential space* because it is normally nonexistent, as the lung adheres to the chest wall by negative pressure. With a tear in the lung tissue, air is pulled into the pleural space. With each breath, more air can accumulate in the pleural space with no place for escape. The pressure increases and at a certain point pushes the heart and great vessels away from the pressure. Respiration is compromised and the ability of the heart to continue to pump blood diminishes. If this process is allowed to continue without treatment, death occurs from hypoxia.

Immediate diagnosis of tension pneumothorax is essential as it can cause death in minutes. It is not an obvious diagnosis, especially in the elder multiple-trauma patient who may have several serious injuries. A high index of suspicion must be maintained in any patient who exhibits any of the following signs after chest wall injury: increasing respiratory difficulty and cyanosis, increasing heart rate, decreasing blood pressure, increasing apprehension and agitation, decreasing movement of the chest wall on the affected side, decreasing breath sounds on auscultation of the chest on the affected side, neck vein distension, and possible subcutaneous emphysema (air beneath the skin).

Hemothorax

Hemothorax occurs after laceration of pulmonary vessels within the thoracic cavity, and is usually a result of penetrating trauma or fractured ribs. Blood accumulates in the pleural space, compromising lung expansion. Rapid accumulation of more than 1500 ml of blood leads to a massive hemothorax. On examination, breath sounds may be diminished, and dullness to percussion may be present on the affected side. The neck veins may be flat from severe hypovolemia or distended because of the mechanical effects of intrathoracic blood. If these findings are present and the patient is in shock, a hemothorax should be suspected.

Cardiac Tamponade

Cardiac tamponade occurs when the pericardial sac becomes filled with blood after trauma. The pericardial sac is a tough tissue that surrounds the heart and is relatively inelastic. After a penetrating or a blunt injury to the anterior chest wall, bleeding can occur, filling this sac. The heart is compressed, causing decreased filling of the heart during diastole. The final result is hypotension as a result of decreased cardiac output. On physical examination, check for hypotension, distended neck veins, and muffled heart tones. If a patient is in shock after chest trauma, with distended neck veins and clear lungs, the prehospital health care provider should suspect cardiac tamponade.

Traumatic Asphyxia

Traumatic asphyxia is a group of symptoms and signs associated with sudden compression of the chest, and sometimes the abdomen. When traumatic asphyxia occurs, the sternum exerts severe pressure on the heart, forcing blood out of the right atrium up into the jugular veins in the neck. On physical exam, look for distended neck veins and a dark blue or purple color of the head, neck, and shoulders. The eyes may be bloodshot and bulging, the tongue and lips may appear swollen and cyanotic, and chest deformity may be present. This is a true emergency requiring immediate transport. Immediate intubation for airway control, or if this is not possible, artificial ventilation with 100 percent oxygen provided through positive pressure, is probably the only way to keep the patient alive during transport.

Other injuries that may not be amenable to immediate intervention but should be considered when deciding the direction of further care are: rib, sternal, or clavicular fractures; pneumothorax or hemothorax; pulmonary or cardiac contusion; disruption of the aorta and great vessels; and rupture of the diaphragm or esophagus. The following injuries are discussed to familiarize the prehospital health care provider with the underlying pathology. Little can be done in the prehospital setting to correct them. Of importance, however, is that suspicion of any of the conditions has an impact on decisions regarding triage, transport time, and information given to the base hospital.

Rib Fractures

Elder patients have weak osteoporotic bones as a result of decreased bone density. Chest wall pain on inspiration or palpation with the history of trauma may indicate a fracture of one or more ribs. The possibility of a pneumothorax or a hemothorax must be considered. The most commonly fractured ribs are those in the bottom half of the rib cage. Bear in mind that rib fractures in this area may indicate a liver or spleen injury. The upper ribs tend to be protected by thick musculature of the upper chest wall. The first two ribs are unusually well protected, and the prehospital health care provider should be aware that fracture of these ribs is associated with aortic and bronchial tears, which can be life threatening. Fractured ribs are painful and the elder patient does not breathe deeply because of pain. Shallow breathing results in alveolar collapse, called *atelectasis.* This less efficient respiratory condition predisposes the elder patient to pneumonia and hypoxia to a greater degree than the younger patient.

Clavicular Fractures

If the clavicle is fractured, the danger is the possibility of injury to the subclavian artery and vein, which lie just beneath the clavicle. With clavicular pain and deformity, the prehospital health care provider must also consider the possibility of a severe chest injury that may require immediate intervention, as previously discussed.

Sternal Fractures

Sternal fracture occurs as a result of direct blunt anterior chest trauma, such as that caused by a steering wheel in a motor vehicle crash. The danger of this fracture is that the heart, which is fragile and may be enlarged in the elder patient, lies beneath the sternum and can be easily lacerated or contused when the sternum is fractured.

Pulmonary Contusion

Pulmonary contusion refers to disruption of the lung tissue with blood and fluid accumulation in the alveoli, the small air sacs in the lung. Intraalveolar edema and tissue inflammation leads to decreased lung compliance and poor ventilation, which causes hypoxia. Pulmonary contusion usually results from a rapid deceleration of the chest, such as in a front-end motor vehicle crash, in which the patient's chest forcefully strikes the steering wheel, and the lung is compressed against the chest wall. Pulmonary contusion, however, is actually less common in elder trauma patients than in younger ones. This is because in younger adults, and pediatric patients in particular, the more compliant chest wall compresses and bruises the lung. In the elder patient, the stiffer rib cage does not compress and usually fractures. The resultant rib fractures can cause frank lacerations of the lung with concomitant pneumothorax or hemothorax. Nevertheless, any significant blow to the chest can cause a pulmonary contusion, and elder patients who have a pulmonary contusion are especially at risk for hypoxia because they have a diminished pulmonary reserve. Pulmonary contusion is usually not evident in the field, because the blood and fluid may take hours to accumulate, but it can become life threatening. In the elder patient, it is important to anticipate the need for intubation and mechanical support before overt respiratory failure occurs.

Cardiac Contusion

Myocardial contusion is a diagnosis for which a high index of suspicion is necessary. As for the younger trauma patient, myocardial contusion usually results from vehicular impact during an automobile accident, particularly one in which the steering column is involved. Certain injuries and symptoms should draw attention to the potential for myocardial contusion, such as rib fractures, sternal fractures, chest wall contusions, pulmonary contusion, chest pain after trauma, new cardiac murmurs, or any signs of cardiac tamponade. The cardiovascular system in elder individuals undergoes many cellular, biochemical, and electrophysiologic changes both from age and disease. This results not only in a decreased cardiac reserve, but also increased rigidity with less adaptability. The heart in the elder patient is also more sensitive to hypoxia and acidosis. There is reduced coronary baseline flow and an impaired coronary response to increased demand. Classic presentation is much like myocardial infarction, with chest pain and radiation to the jaw and arm. However, the elder patient does not always manifest classic signs and symptoms, especially if they are diabetic and have diminished cardiac sensitivity. Elder patients with cardiac contusion may present without any other symptoms except shock, so a high index of suspicion is mandatory when evaluating these patients. The rhythm strip may show dysrhythmias and conduction blocks. Treatment of arrhythmias resulting from cardiac contusion is done according to standard ACLS protocols.

Tracheobronchial Injuries

Injuries of the trachea and bronchi should be suspected with any injury of the upper chest in which the patient has significant difficulty breathing, continues to cough, or has associated hemoptysis (coughing up blood). Often there is subcutaneous emphysema. This injury can be a result of either blunt or penetrating trauma. Compression of a hyperinflated chest causes a phenomenon called the *paper bag syndrome*. As the driver sees the impending impact, he or she takes a deep gasp of air and holds it. During the crash, the chest impacts on the steering wheel or dashboard and compresses the hyperinflated thorax against a closed glottis. The trachea and bronchus rupture like a sealed paper bag between two clapping hands. Subcutaneous emphysema, pneumothorax, and hypoxia can result.

Disruption of the Aorta and Great Vessels

Tears of the aorta and great vessels occur with significant deceleration and blunt injuries to the chest. High-speed vehicular crashes and falls from great heights are the most common causes. Eighty-five percent of patients die at the scene because these injuries can cause immediate and total loss of cardiac output. The other 15 percent must be treated quickly at the hospital. The prehospital health care provider should recognize the mechanisms of injury that could result in injury to the great vessels. Patients, if awake, may relate anterior chest pain, back pain, and particularly intrascapular pain. There may be shortness of breath and difficulty swallowing because of compression on the trachea and esophagus from an expanding hematoma. Hoarseness can result from compression of the recurrent laryngeal nerve, which wraps around the aorta. Hypotension often occurs because of obstruction of blood flow through the torn area. There may be a discrepancy in the blood pressure of the left and right arm from decreased blood flow to one side. The elder patient may have evidence of a left hemothorax, which occurs if the bleeding ruptures out into the left chest from the mediastinum. The elder heart and great vessels are structurally less resilient than in younger people. A reduction in elasticity and an increase in the calcium content of the great vessels leads to increased rigidity and less adaptability. Tearing of the intima (the innermost tissue lining the aorta) at the site of atherosclerotic plaque may cause an aortic dissection or traumatic aneurysm. Although complete transection typically results in immediate death, the occasional patient maintains adequate perfusion throughout an incompletely transected aorta to survive to presentation in the emergency department. A high index of suspicion on the part of the prehospital health care providers based on the mechanism of injury is critical. These injuries are repairable only if immediately recognized and treated by the hospital personnel.

Rupture of the Diaphragm and Esophagus

The diaphragm divides the chest and the abdomen by means of a sheet of muscle. A tear in this structure results in the intestinal contents herniating into the chest. Field presentation may include respiratory distress and shock. The rupture usually occurs on the left side because the liver, which lies just below the diaphragm on the right side, protects the right side of the diaphragm. Consequently, decreased breath sounds and at times even bowel sounds can be heard in the left chest. Rupture of the esophagus is a difficult diagnosis even in the hospital setting. Elder patients often do not manifest signs of tissue irritation, and may complain of only vague chest discomfort, making the diagnosis even more difficult.

ASSESSMENT

Assessment of chest trauma begins with the initial assessment (ABCs). The goal of initial assessment is to detect and correct any immediate threats to the patient's life. This should be followed by a thorough focused assessment (complete history and physical examination). Start by evaluating the mechanism of injury carefully, which suggests the probability of chest injury. Important details about the mechanism of injury are listed in Table 13.3.

First, the Airway should be assessed for patency. The presence of snoring or gurgling may indicate potential problems with the airway. Second, the adequacy of Breathing should be determined. Look for spontaneous rise and fall of the chest with respiration rate of 12–18 breaths per minute. The chest wall should be observed for any area of asymmetrical movement that may suggest a flail chest. If the patient's airway is compromised or the patient is not breathing spontaneously, open the airway by using the head–tilt/chin lift or jaw-thrust maneuver. Check for dentures and if loose or broken, remove them. Always maintain stabilization of the cervical spine in all trauma patients. Once the airway is patent, reevaluate the status of breathing by observing the spontaneous rise and fall of the chest wall. Use airway adjuncts (oropharyngeal airway or nasopharyngeal airway if no facial trauma is evident) and a ventilatory device such as bag–valve mask as needed. Circulation: look for signs of hypovolemia, such as rapid and weak peripheral pulses, cool clammy

Table 13.3. Blunt Trauma

Motor Vehicle Crash
    Estimated speed of both vehicles on impact.
    Orientation of the vehicles (e.g., head-on, broadside)
    Trajectory and extent of damage to patient's vehicle.
    Was there an explosion or fire?
    Was the patient restrained, and did an air bag deploy?
    Were the windshield, dashboard, and steering wheel intact?
    Was there a loss of consciousness prior to or after the crash?
    Were there any prescription medications, drugs, or alcohol recovered from the patient or car?
    How long did it take to extricate the patient?
    What is the ambient temperature (elder patients are easily prone to hypothermia)?

Fall
    Estimated height?
    Possible reason for fall (e.g., electrocution, explosion).
    Was there an initial loss of consciousness at the scene?
    Were there any prescription medications, drugs, or alcohol recovered from the patient or scene?
    How long was the patient down?
    What is the ambient temperature?

Penetrating Trauma—Stab or gunshot wound
    Description of the weapon (e.g., length, width, caliber)
    Were there any prescription medications, drugs, or alcohol recovered from the patient?
    How long was the patient down?

skin, poor capillary refill, and diminished level of consciousness. These signs and symptoms may mean that there is an internal blood loss within the chest cavity. Quickly expose the patient by removing or cutting off clothing, especially any constricting garments around the chest and neck.

Focused assessment follows completion of the initial assessment and correction of any immediate threats to the patient's life. This should begin with a brief history of the current problem using the mnemonic SAMPLE: Signs and symptoms, Allergies, Medications, Past medical history, Last oral intake, and Events leading to the injury. Ask the patient where they have discomfort, or about other symptoms. Ask the patient about any allergies to medications, foods, or environmental factors, and always look for a medical alert tag. Identify any medications the patient is taking. Ask for pertinent medical history including recent or past medical problems, surgeries, and injuries. Get specific information about the last oral intake, including the time and quantity of both solid and liquid food. Finally, identify the events leading to the injury (to help clarify the mechanism of injury and understand the potential force involved).

Next, prepare to do a complete physical examination. Use the acronym DCAP-BTLS to remember the eight components of a thorough examination. *Deformities* occur when bones are broken, causing an abnormal position or shape. *Contusions* are bruises. *Abrasions* occur when the top layers of the skin are scraped away. *Penetrations* or *Punctures* involve when an object penetrates the skin, such as gunshot wound or stab wound. *Burns* can result from exposure to heat, chemicals, electricity, or radiation. *Tenderness* is sensitivity to touch. *Lacerations* are cuts in the surface of the skin. *Swelling* is a response of the body to traumatic injury and makes the area look larger than usual. Use the head-to-toe order of assessment, starting at the patient's head. In chest trauma patients, it is important to examine the neck for jugular vein distension. The jugular veins are large veins on both sides of the neck. Distended jugular veins signify increased pressure in the cardiopulmonary system. Inspect and palpate the chest for DCAP-BTLS. Contusions or abrasions over the chest wall indicate an increased risk of cardiopulmonary injury, especially elder patients, because of loss of elasticity and increased chest wall rigidity. Also evaluate the chest for paradoxical motion and crepitation. Paradoxical motion is movement of part of the chest wall in the opposite direction from the rest of the chest wall during inhalation and exhalation. Think of a flail chest when paradoxical motion is seen. *Crepitation* is the sound and feel of broken bones or air underneath the skin, and can indicate rib fractures or critical organ injury.

Evaluate the chest by feeling the clavicles first. Palpate the sternum and the entire rib cage for crepitation. Place one hand on each side of the patient's rib cage to assess for paradoxical motion. Use a stethoscope in the apices (top of the chest) at the mid-clavicular line, and at the bases at the mid-axillary line, bilaterally, to determine if breath sounds are present, diminished, or absent. Determine if breath sounds are present bilaterally and if they are equal. The respiratory rate should be accurately determined. A respiratory rate of less than 10 or greater than 29 is an indication for transfer to a trauma receiving facility. A decrease or increase in the respiratory rate is one of the earliest indicators of respiratory distress and significant chest injury. Look for use of the accessory muscles, which is characterized by intercostal retractions, suprasternal retractions, and use of abdominal muscles. Twenty percent of patients with a pneumothorax have a severe paroxysm of coughing associated with the onset of the pneumothorax. Apprehension and fear are often present and may be the result of hypoxia. Diaphoresis is also commonly present.

One of the biggest pitfalls in evaluating and managing the elder patient is that commonly used parameters such as vital signs to assess hemodynamic status can be misleading. In the elder patient, a tachycardic response may be blunted by medications (beta-blockers, calcium-channel blockers), intrinsic conduction disease, or decreased responsiveness of the elder heart to catecholamines, which are normally released during stressful events. Thus, tachycardia cannot always be used as a reliable early sign of internal hemorrhage. Blood pressure also can be misleading because elder persons generally have an elevated blood pressure when compared with younger persons. A systolic blood pressure of 110 mmHg may actually be hypotensive for a person who normally has a systolic blood pressure of 160 mmHg or greater. Mental status may be difficult to assess in the patient with underlying dementia. Elder patients also have an altered perception of pain, making them unaware of potential injuries. It is crucial for the prehospital health care provider to look beyond the chief complaint when assessing the elder patient with chest trauma. In one study, more than 25 percent of elder patients presenting with one chief complaint suggesting only one injury were discovered to have a second injury. The difficulty and the challenge for health care providers is that elder trauma patients are intolerant of shock for even a brief amount of time, yet routine clinical parameters are often unreliable.

RETURNING TO THE CASE

This patient obviously has a severe chest injury. He has rib fractures and may have a pneumothorax or hemothorax (or both) as well as cardiac tamponade. He is also at risk for a flail chest, which may be difficult to detect because of his splinting of respirations. After he is moved into the ambulance, he develops severe respiratory distress and tracheal deviation to the right.

(continued)

His neck veins are distended. His blood pressure drops to 80/40. You recognize a tension pneumothorax and quickly place a large-bore needle in the second intercostal space in the mid-clavicular line. There is an immediate rush of air and with ventilatory assistance, the patient becomes less tachycardic and tachypneic. Breath sounds are now present, but still diminished on the left. His blood pressure improves and his neck veins return to normal. You observe paradoxical respirations on the left side and place direct pressure on that area to improve the patient's respiratory effort and diminish his discomfort. You transport him rapidly to the hospital.

STABILIZATION/TREATMENT

The priorities for out of hospital care should be directed toward maintaining the airway and preventing further injury. Airway obstruction is generally recognized as the most rapidly fatal problem. Elder trauma patients are much more likely to have dentures or other materials in their mouths that could lead to partial or complete airway obstruction. Intubate early any elder patient who is unable to protect their airway. Particular attention should be directed toward immobilizing the cervical spine in any injury remotely suggesting a cervical spine injury to prevent any further damage. Many elder patients already have underlying degenerative disease such as arthritis. Oxygen supplementation is almost universally indicated because the elder patient often has underlying cardiac or respiratory disease with a limited cardiovascular reserve. If the patient exhibits any early signs of shock, begin fluid resuscitation with two large-bore IVs. Consider pneumatic anti-shock garment (PASG) application according to local protocols. Thermal protection must also be a high priority because elder patients are much more prone to hypothermia (as a result of loss of body mass and impaired temperature regulation) than younger patients.

The initial assessment and rapid trauma assessment should be completed within 2 min of the prehospital health care provider's arrival at the scene. The critically injured elder patient should be transported to the appropriate trauma receiving facility if any life-threatening signs or symptoms are present. Time must be devoted to only those procedures that make a difference in the patient's outcome. After the primary and secondary assessment has been completed, specific treatment of chest injury should be initiated in the field.

Flail Chest

Treatment of a flail chest in the field depends on the degree of respiratory distress. If the patient is awake and able to verbalize that he is breathing easily, stabilization of the segment using a bulky dressing taped to the chest may be sufficient. In certain cases, when cervical spine trauma has been excluded, the patient can be turned onto the side of the flail segment, so that the flail segment is stabilized by the stretcher or backboard. If there is a bilateral flail or flail of the sternum, then this maneuver is of no help. Simply placing one's hands over the flail segment and keeping the floating ribs from moving outward may help temporarily. If there is severe respiratory distress with a flail chest associated with cyanosis and decreased mental status, then intubation with positive-pressure ventilation is required. If intubation is unsuccessful, then initial use of high-flow oxygen and a bag–valve mask device may be used until intubation in the emergency department is performed.

Tension Pneumothorax

This is a serious life-threatening insult to the cardiorespiratory system. Treatment of a tension pneumothorax requires the creation of an opening through which air from the pleural space is allowed to escape. Look for signs and symptoms, such as unequal breath sounds, agitation, cyanosis, lethargy, and jugular vein distention with increasing dyspnea.

Decompression can be performed with a large-gauge catheter-over-needle, preferably 14 gauge or larger, placed in the second intercostal space in the mid-clavicular line on the affected side. The overlying skin should first be prepped with betadine or alcohol. When the catheter enters the pleural space, a rush of air is heard. Often improvement is noticed immediately in the patient. The needle is withdrawn, and the catheter can be left in place with a flutter valve so that air can flow from the chest but not into the chest. A finger cot with the end cut off and fastened to the catheter serves the need. If the catheter is removed, the procedure can be repeated if indicated during transport.

Traumatic Asphyxia, Cardiac Tamponade, and Massive Hemothorax

Treatment in the field usually consists of rapidly transporting the patient to the hospital, where the pericardial sac is drained either by placing a catheter into the sac or by opening the chest and directly draining and stopping the bleeding. Establish two large-bore IVs, provide supplemental oxygen or intubate as necessary, and place the patient on a cardiac monitor. Transport to hospital as soon as possible following primary resuscitation guidelines.

Open Chest Wounds

When faced with a patient with poor respirations and an open chest wound, immediately treat the wound with a semi-occlusive dressing.

Tape the dressing on top of the wound and make sure that it is at least 2 inches wider than the wound on all sides. Leave one corner of the dressing unsealed, creating a valve, which relieves pressure in the thoracic cavity. As the patient inhales, the dressing seals the wound. During exhalation, the free corner acts as a flutter valve to release air that is trapped in the thoracic cavity. Administer a high concentration of oxygen. Great diligence must be maintained to ensure that a tension pneumothorax does not develop as a result of this closure. Closure of an open sucking chest wound usually improves the patient's ability to breathe, as better bellows action is permitted. This is because a large wound can prevent the development of negative pleural pressure and result in an inability of the lung to draw in air as the chest wall expands.

If an object is found to be impaled in the chest, do not remove it. Cover the corner of the entry wound with an occlusive and bulky dressing. Completely stabilize the object so it will not move or dislodge during transport. Removal of the object may cause internal bleeding and lead to shock.

Rib Fractures

Always render care for possible rib fractures. This helps reduce the patient's pain and protects the lungs and vessels that are underneath the ribs. To provide care for possible fractured ribs, place the forearm of the injured side in a sling across the patient's chest. A swathe can be applied to support the arm. Follow special protocols for pain management using narcotics. Pain relief often improves ventilatory effort, but narcotic administration can also cause respiratory depression, especially in the elder patient, so careful monitoring of the patient's respiratory status by the prehospital health care provider is mandatory.

Tracheobronchial Injuries

In the field, proper airway and ventilatory support suffices until the patient is transported to the hospital. If intubation is attempted in the field, ventilation may not be improved if the tear is at or near the level of the carina where the bronchi divide from the trachea, where most tears occur. In this situation, expeditious transport to the hospital is indicated.

Cardiac and Pulmonary Contusions

This type of injury requires rapid transport to the hospital after the airway has been secured. Administer supplemental oxygen, establish two large-bore IVs if possible, and place the patient on a cardiac monitor. Implement standard ACLS protocols if arrhythmias develop.

Aortic and Great Vessel Injury

Field care demands immediate transportation to the hospital after the airway has been secured and supplemental oxygen administered. Two large-bore IVs should be established, but should not slow the transfer. Patients with aortic or great vessel injuries are frequently unstable. Many die at the scene of the injury. Finally, for both diaphragmatic and esophageal injuries, diagnosis is not possible in the field, and transport to the hospital is the immediate indicated action after initial and focused assessments.

CASE OUTCOME

After arrival in the emergency department, the patient received a left chest tube that revealed only a small hemothorax. A chest x-ray showed that the pneumothorax had improved, and a cardiac echo showed no tamponade. He had a small flail segment involving two ribs on the left, but no other significant injuries were found. He was given narcotics for pain control and was admitted to the trauma intensive care unit for aggressive pulmonary care. He did not require intubation and was discharged home on the sixth hospital day.

CONCLUSION

Although the overall mortality rate for the elder patient with multiple injuries is about 20 percent, and although some who survive the initial trauma require long-term care, the majority of survivors are able to return to a satisfactory quality of life. Favorable outcomes depend on rapid evaluation by prehospital personnel, careful identification of mechanism of injury, aggressive treatment of injuries, diligent monitoring, and prevention of pulmonary and septic complications. Injury to the chest accounts for a very high percentage of traumatic deaths. The prehospital health care provider should have a high index of suspicion for injury to this region and prepare for aggressive intervention. Careful attention to the mechanism of injury and force involved assists hospital personnel who also care for these patients. Identifying the effects of trauma from baseline disease can be extremely complex, thus giving the prehospital health care provider the challenge of the initial assessment and management and the opportunity to reduce the patient's morbidity and mortality.

REVIEW QUESTIONS

1. Most elder patients with chest trauma
   a. die at the scene of the injury
   b. require life-saving operative intervention
   c. survive with rapid prehospital intervention and supportive care
   d. require immediate intubation

2. All of the following are chest injuries requiring immediate intervention in the field *except*
   a. pulmonary contusion
   b. tension pneumothorax
   c. traumatic asphyxia
   d. flail chest

3. Elders are more likely than younger people to have rib fractures as a result of blunt chest trauma because
   a. their chest walls are more compliant
   b. most have kyphosis, which causes the chest wall to be stiff and more brittle
   c. in elders, more force is transmitted to the ribs during a chest injury
   d. most elders have osteoporosis

4. The best way to successfully detect a flail chest in an elder patient is
   a. palpation of the chest to feel for the flail segment
   b. auscultation of the chest to detect diminished breath sounds
   c. only by x-ray; flail chest cannot be detected accurately in the field
   d. observing the chest wall motion during breathing

5. All of the following are signs of cardiac tamponade in the elder patient with blunt chest trauma *except*
   a. hypotension
   b. muffled heart tones
   c. jugular venous distension
   d. diminished breath sounds on the affected side

6. The elder patient with suspected fractures to the lower half of the rib cage after blunt trauma is especially at risk for
   a. flail chest
   b. liver or spleen injury, which may result in sudden shock
   c. hemothorax
   d. tension pneumothorax

7. All are important details to learn at the scene of a motor vehicle crash involving an elder person *except*
   a. estimated speed and trajectory of the vehicles at the time of impact
   b. previous underlying medical conditions or medications taken
   c. whether the patient has had prior crashes
   d. extrication time

8. All are reasons that it may be difficult to detect impending shock in the elder patients with chest trauma *except*
   a. they may have had a previous myocardial infarction
   b. they may not get tachycardic because of underlying conduction disease of the heart
   c. they may be bradycardic because of the use of beta-blockers
   d. they may be in the early stages of shock even when the blood pressure is normal, for example, 110/60

9. The correct prehospital placement of a 14-gauge needle into the chest of an elder patient with suspected tension pneumothorax is
   a. under the second rib in the mid-calvicular line
   b. in the second intercostal space in the mid-axillary line
   c. in the second intercostal space in the mid-clavicular line, over the rib
   d. in the fifth intercostal space in the mid-clavicular line

10. All of the following are true about open chest wounds in the elder patient *except*
    a. a valve should be created with 1-inch margins around the wound to minimize the risk of a tension pneumothorax
    b. impaled objects should be left in place
    c. patients may rapidly develop a tension pneumothorax
    d. patients may require intubation even after a flutter valve is created

SUGGESTED READING

Alexander, R. H. and H. J. Proctor, 1993. *Advanced trauma life support.* 5th ed. Chicago: American College of Surgeons.

14

Abdominal and Pelvic Trauma

Selim Suner, MD, MS

OBJECTIVES

By the end of this chapter, the prehospital health care provider should be able to:

1 Identify the specific epidemiology of abdominal and pelvic trauma in elders.

2 Provide initial evaluation and treatment considerations of abdominal and pelvic trauma in elders.

3 Describe the pitfalls in the evaluation and management of abdominal and pelvic trauma in elders.

CASE

You are called to the apartment of an elder woman who fell down in the bathtub and could not get up. When you arrive at the scene, she is sitting on the edge of the toilet, is pale, and states that her stomach hurts when she breathes. Her daughter is with her, and states that she was fixing dinner for her mother when she heard a crash in the bathroom. She found the patient crumpled against the side of the bathtub, and helped her up. The patient is alert and oriented times three and denies loss of consciousness. She holds her left side throughout your examination and occasionally groans in pain. Her vital signs are blood pressure 110/60, heart rate 90, and respiratory rate of 22. Her pulse oximetry is 98 percent and cardiac monitoring shows normal sinus rhythm. You place her on supplemental oxygen, start a large-bore IV, and fully immobilize her cervical spine. What do you think is the problem with this woman? What additional history should you ask for? Is she in danger? What out-of-hospital stabilization and treatment should you initiate prior to hospital transfer?

EPIDEMIOLOGY

Up to 35 percent of elder patients with multiple trauma have significant injuries to the abdomen. These injuries increase the risk of mortality rate in the elder population five-fold compared to younger patients with similar injuries.

The major mechanisms of trauma that cause injury to the abdomen and pelvis of elder patients are falls, motor vehicle crashes, pedestrians being hit, gunshot wounds, and stab wounds. The incidence of falls and being struck by a vehicle is higher in elders compared those under 65 years of age. Although the incidence of other mechanisms of abdominal and pelvic trauma is lower in the elder patient than in younger patients, the morbidity and mortality is greater in elders. Only motorcycle crashes, which are more prevalent in the younger age group, have the same mortality for young and old. In one study, the incidence of falls was 46 percent for elder patients with abdominal trauma, and the overall mortality was 12 percent. For pedestrians hit, the incidence of elderly patients with abdominal trauma was 10 percent and mortality was 33 percent in this age group. For penetrating trauma, the incidence was 8 percent for elders compared to 24 percent for younger patients. The mortality from penetrating trauma was more than 50 percent for gunshot wounds and 17 percent for stab wounds in the elder population. For motorcycle crashes the incidence in young trauma patients was 20 times that for elder patients but the mortality rate was the same for both groups of patients at 12 percent. The issue of falls in elders is covered in detail in the musculoskeletal trauma chapter. Motor vehicle crashes accounted for 5000 deaths in the elder age group in 1989. Failure to use safety belts and alcohol use are major contributing risk factors for abdominal and pelvic trauma from motor vehicle crashes in the elder population. Also, because of decreased cognition and perception and diminished reaction times, elder pedestrians are at higher risk of being struck by motor vehicles. The incidence of penetrating trauma among elders in urban areas is growing.

In one study, the factors that were associated with mortality in elder patients with abdominal or pelvic trauma were previous heart attack, kidney disease, need for ventilatory or cardiovascular support, or a systolic blood pressure below 90 mmHg on admission to the hospital. Most deaths occurred within the first 24 hr.

INITIAL EVALUATION AND TREATMENT CONSIDERATIONS

The principles of evaluating the elder patient with abdominal or pelvic trauma are completing the initial assessment by assuring the patency of the airway, adequate respiration, and hemodynamic stability. In this chapter, particular attention is directed to the abdomen, pelvis, and genitalia during the focused assessment, but the prehospital health care provider should always bear in mind that the abdomen may be only one of multiple injured areas in the elder trauma victim. First, the disrobed abdomen is inspected for distension, bruising, abrasions, lacerations, puncture wounds, and penetrating foreign bodies. Ostomy sites and bags should be inspected for contents. The presence of blood should be noted. The patient should be log-rolled to examine the flank and back. Finally, the abdomen and flank are palpated and areas of tenderness, rebound tenderness, and referred pain are noted. The genitalia should be inspected for bleeding or foreign body.

All elder patients with abdominal trauma should be monitored closely during the evaluation and transport phases of their care. Administration of supplemental oxygen, large-bore IV access, cardiac monitoring, continuous pulse oximetry, and frequent vital sign measurements are essential.

After the initial and focused assessments, treatment should be initiated immediately for shock, including suspected intra-abdominal bleeding. Obtain intravenous access with at least one 16-gauge or larger bore catheters and an infuse normal saline or lactated ringer's solution. Establish two IV lines [with the second one at keep vein open (KVO)] in case the patient deteriorates during stabilization or transport. Elevate the lower extremities and warm the patient with prewarmed blankets and fluids, if possible. The ambulance environment should also be prewarmed to minimize heat loss in the elderly patient. The use of the pneumatic anti-shock garment (PASG) is controversial in the management of trauma, but it should be considered if local protocols call for its use for patients in shock. Vasopressor medications should be considered, but only after volume replacement has been adequately achieved in the elder patient with abdominal or pelvic trauma. Some prehospital systems have been using colloidal fluids such as hetastarch and blood substitute agents for persons in shock. The use of these agents, in accordance with local protocols, for elder patients in shock may also be appropriate. If transport times are expected to be long, early elective intubation and assisted oxygenation and ventilation should be considered for elder patients in persistent shock. Because elders have a higher ventilation perfusion mismatch (more "dead space" in the lungs), shock often causes severe hypoxia and further hinders tissue oxygenation. If the patient is being intubated electively, use of induction agents that cause significant hypotension, such as sodium pentothal, midazolam, and lorazepam should not be used or used with extreme caution, particularly if the patient is already in shock, and only under the direction of medical control.

Eviscerated abdominal contents should be covered with a sterile sheet or abdominal bandage moistened with warmed sterile saline. Particular attention should be paid to maintaining a warm environment, as evisceration leads to increased heat loss.

Any foreign body penetrating the abdomen or perineum should be left in place and not pulled out in the field, because such action may lead to increased bleeding and further injury. Care should be taken to immobilize foreign objects prior to transportation or movement of patient in order to prevent further harm.

Most causes of intra-abdominal bleeding from blunt trauma are the same for elder and younger patients. Injury to the right upper quadrant of the abdomen may cause lacerations of the liver. Left upper quadrant abdominal injury may injure the spleen, resulting in intra-abdominal hemorrhage. Blunt trauma may also cause injury to the kidneys, pancreas, and bowels. Injury to these organs is less likely to cause immediate bleeding and shock. In penetrating trauma, bleeding from large vessels such as the vena cava, aorta, major branches of the aorta, or bleeding from the solid organs may cause shock. Unlike young persons, hemorrhage in the retroperitoneum (in the flank areas, behind the abdominal cavity) from blunt trauma is a cause of significant hemorrhage in elders. It is thought that loss of tissue turgor (tightness) in elders may contribute to unabated retroperitoneal hemorrhage by preventing local tamponade of the hematoma. Elder persons taking oral anticoagulant medications such as warfarin or aspirin are at particular risk for retroperitoneal hemorrhage.

RETURNING TO THE CASE

While loading the patient into the ambulance, she complains of severe pain. You recheck her vital signs and find that her blood pressure is now 70 by palpation, with a heart rate of 140. You give her a 500 cc IV bolus of normal saline and start a second large-bore IV. This patient probably has a splenic laceration. You ask her about medical history and current medications. You find out that she has a history of hypertension and takes hydrochlorothiazide and a beta blocker. These medications may obscure the signs of early shock, as they did in this patient. An initial blood pressure of 110/70 is not always reassuring in an elder patient with a history of hypertension. You should also ask whether she takes blood thinners, such as warfarin (Coumadin®), because this would make a patient with a splenic laceration more likely to deteriorate quickly. You recognize that the patient is critically injured, and transport her immediately to the emergency department.

PITFALLS IN THE EVALUATION AND MANAGEMENT OF ABDOMINAL AND PELVIC TRAUMA IN ELDERS

The major reason for the increased mortality and morbidity elders suffer from trauma compared to their younger counterparts is because the elder person's cardiovascular system is unable to respond to the increased demand brought about by the injury. Elders are less able to increase their cardiac output, which is the product of heart rate and the amount of blood pumped with each heartbeat. Elder hearts are also more susceptible to arrhythmias. This tendency arises from a stiffer heart muscle and the difficulty elders have in increasing oxygen delivery to the heart in response to heightened demand. The use of beta-blockers, diuretics, and calcium-channel blockers are more common in elders. These medications further diminish the cardiovascular response to trauma and blood loss.

In addition to impaired cardiovascular supply, the kidneys of elder patients are also ill equipped to meet the demands of trauma. The elder person's renal function is often diminished, so that the kidneys are unable to concentrate urine properly. This often leads to dehydration.

Watching for telltail signs of bleeding and shock, such as tachycardia, vasoconstriction, diminished urine output, tachypnea, narrowed pulse pressure, and altered mental status is much less reliable in elder victims of trauma with suspected abdominal or pelvic injury. In one study, the vital signs of the elder patient did not accurately predict the seriousness of the injury.

It is common for elder patients with occult abdominal injury and bleeding to be in unrecognized normotensive shock. This happens when the patient's baseline blood pressure is elevated, and after trauma, the blood pressure falls into the normal range as a result of internal hemorrhage and shock. Do not be reassured if the elder patient's blood pressure and pulse are normal after abdominal or pelvic trauma as this may be the first sign of shock. Monitor vital signs continuously and closely, always establish an IV lifeline, and be prepared to resuscitate! The key to proper management of these patients is prompt completion of the primary and secondary survey, initiation of basic treatment for shock and hasty transport to a hospital emergency department. When dealing with the injured elder patient, the prehospital provider should remember that no elder trauma patient is stable, and that every minute is golden.

CASE OUTCOME

The patient arrives in the emergency department with a blood pressure of 100/50. She has an abdominal CT scan that shows a ruptured spleen. No chest or extremity injuries are found. She is taken emergently to the operating room for a splenectomy. Her hospital course is complicated by the development of pneumonia, but she is discharged home after a 2-week stay.

REVIEW QUESTIONS

1. What percentage of elder patients with multiple trauma have significant injuries of the abdomen or pelvis?
   a. 15 percent
   b. 35 percent
   c. 50 percent
   d. 85 percent

2. Elder patients with abdominal or pelvic trauma
   a. have a higher rate of morbidity than younger patients with abdominal or pelvic trauma
   b. have a higher rate of mortality than younger patients with abdominal or pelvic trauma
   c. have a higher rate of morbidity and mortality than younger patients with abdominal or pelvic trauma
   d. have lower rates of mortality than young patients with abdominal trauma

3. All of the following increase the risk of mortality in the elder patient with abdominal or pelvic trauma *except*
   a. previous heart attack
   b. diabetes
   c. kidney disease
   d. need for ventilatory support

4. Prehospital management of elder patients with penetrating abdominal trauma that has caused eviscerated abdominal contents includes all *except*
   a. removal of the penetrating foreign body
   b. stabilization of the penetrating foreign body
   c. covering eviscerated abdominal contents with a dressing moistened with normal saline
   d. minimizing the patient's heat loss

5. Elder patients with blunt abdominal trauma are more likely than younger patients to have
   a. injury to the bowel
   b. injury to the liver
   c. injury to the pancreas
   d. retroperitoneal hematoma

6. All are reasons for increased mortality in the elder population after abdominal or pelvic trauma *except*
   a. elders have a higher rate of cardiac arrhythmias
   b. elders are less able to increase their cardiac output
   c. elders are more likely to have injuries to the aorta or vena cava
   d. elders are often taking beta-blockers or calcium-channel blockers

7. The easiest mistake the prehospital provider can make in the field with an elder patient suffering from abdominal or pelvic trauma is
   a. elective intervention for persistent shock
   b. failure to recognize that the patient is taking warfarin (Coumadin®)
   c. failure to use the pneumatic anti-shock garment
   d. failure to recognize that a normal blood pressure may indicate early shock

8. All are contributing risk factors for abdominal trauma in the elder patient *except*
   a. air bag deployment in a motor vehicle crash
   b. alcohol intoxication
   c. not using seatbelts
   d. decreased reaction time

SUGGESTED READING

ATLS Advanced Truma Life Support Program for Doctors, 6th ed. 1997. Chicago: American College of Surgeons.

Aucar, J. A. and K. L. Mattox, 1998. Trauma. Chapter 33 in R. B. Adkins Jr. and H. W. Scott Jr., *Surgical care in the elderly*, 2d ed. Philadelpia: Lippincott–Raven, pp. 531–565.

15

Musculoskeletal Trauma

Selim Suner, MD, MS

OBJECTIVES

By the end of this chapter, the prehospital health care provider should be able to:

1 Understand the specific epidemiology of musculoskeletal trauma in the elder patient.

2 Describe the initial evaluation and treatment considerations in elder musculoskeletal trauma.

3 Review commonly seen fractures in elders.

4 Be familiar with fracture prevention in elders.

CASE

You are called to a nursing home. An elder man fell on the way to the bathroom and was found on the floor, moaning in pain. He responds to you verbally and appears to be alert but disoriented. The staff tell you that he's "out to lunch" and that's his baseline. They do not think he experienced a loss of consciousness. They heard a thud and he cried out. A staff nurse arrived in the room a few moments later to find him on the floor. When they attempted to stand him up, he complained about his leg, so they returned him to the floor. His blood pressure is 170/100, his heart rate is 45 and irregular, and his respiratory rate is 22. Initial and focused assessments reveal a contusion on the occipital scalp, mild neck tenderness, and a right leg that is foreshortened and externally rotated. What do you think is the problem with this man? What additional questions should you ask the patient or the nursing home staff? Is he in danger? What additional treatment can you offer him? Are there any medications you should consider giving him? If so, what are the appropriate dosages?

EPIDEMIOLOGY

The proportion of elders in the U.S. population is increasing as the life expectancy increases as a result of better health care and a more health conscious population. Currently, 12.5 percent of the U.S. population is older than 65. By the year 2030, this proportion will increase to 20 percent. Successful treatment of musculoskeletal injuries, particularly fractures, in elder patients involves many parts of the health care system, including effective prehospital care, emergency medicine, orthopedics, rehabilitation, psychiatry, and social work. These injuries have a large economic impact on the health care system. Appropriate treatment has an impact on the quality of life of the patient and may also be life saving.

Predisposing Factors to Fractures in Elders

Both intrinsic and extrinsic factors contribute to musculoskeletal trauma in elders. Intrinsic factors such as osteoporosis and stress fractures arise from physiologic changes of aging bone. Extrinsic factors including falls and motor vehicle crashes are more common in elder patients because of changes in vision, balance, coordination, reaction time, use of multiple medications, and the effects of chronic illness.

Osteoporosis. *Osteoporosis* is the most common age-related bone disease, defined as an absolute decrease in bone density. The remaining bone structure is normal. Twenty percent of cases of osteoporosis are the result of other disease states such as cancer and endocrine disorders or may be associated with certain drugs such as steroids, anticonvulsants, and alcohol. The remaining cases are a result of aging. There are two types of osteoporosis. Type I osteoporosis is seen in women after menopause and is related to the decline in production of the hormone estrogen. Fractures of the distal radius and vertebral body compression fractures are the most common fractures associated with type I osteoporosis. Type II osteoporosis is seen in both men and women over the age of 50 and is a progressive slow rate of bone loss. The most common fractures associated with type II osteoporosis are hip fractures and wedge fractures of the vertebral body (resulting in a *dorsal kyphosis,* or curvature of the spine). *Osteoporosis is the most important clinical risk factor for fracture in elders.*

Pathological fractures. *Pathological fractures* are fractures that occur in bone whose integrity is compromised by a disease process within one part of the bone. The most common causes of pathological fractures are metastatic cancers and Paget's disease. Breast, lung, kidney, thyroid, and prostate cancers commonly spread to bone. Approximately 10 percent of patients with these metastases sustain fractures. In addition to metastatic cancer, primary cancers of the blood, such as multiple myeloma, lymphoma, and leukemia, and less commonly, tumors of the bone such as osteosarcoma and chondrosarcoma, can cause fractures.

Paget's disease is a pathological increase in bone turnover characterized by breakdown of normal bone and deposition of abnormal bone. Paget's disease is more prevalent in the elder population, although it is also seen in younger people. Ten percent to thirty percent of patients with Paget's disease sustain pathological fractures. Often these fractures are the presenting manifestation, of Paget's disease.

Stress fractures. Although commonly thought of as a disease of athletic young people, stress fractures are also common in the elder population. Stress fractures in elders are seen after foot surgery, total knee replacement, and total hip replacement. These fractures occur because of increased weight bearing and use of joints after a period of immobilization. Stress fractures in elders are most commonly seen in women with rheumatoid arthritis.

Falls. Every year, about one-third of the elder population experience a fall, and half of those who fall sustain a significant injury. Women are twice as susceptible to falls and sustain more serious injuries. Seventy-five percent of deaths secondary to falls occur in the elder population. Ten percent to twenty-five percent of nursing home patients sustain a fall each year.

Hip fractures, the most serious musculoskeletal complication of falls, occur in 1 percent of patients who fall. Five percent of falls result in other fractures, 10 percent result in other serious injury, and 50 percent of falls cause minor soft tissue injury requiring no medical attention.

There are multiple factors that contribute to the cause of falls in elders. Falls may be the result of underlying medical conditions. Thirty percent of falls result from sudden weakness of the legs without loss of consciousness (drop attack). Syncope (fainting), strokes, transient ischemic attacks (TIA), seizures, poor eyesight, orthostatic hypotension, and loss of balance are some other conditions that may cause falls in elders.

Medication use is also associated with falls in elders. Although combinations of drugs are more commonly implicated in falls in elders, the use of barbiturates, phenothiazines, tricyclic antidepressants, benzodiazepines, antihypertensives, and diuretics may cause falls.

There are also many environmental factors that contribute to falls in elders. Nearly half of all falls are a result of extrinsic environmental factors. Stairs; inadequate lighting; carpet edges; throw rugs; slippery floors; electrical cords; inappropriate bed, chair, and toilet seat heights; use of high-heel shoes; and wheelchair use in nursing homes are some of the environmental factors associated with falls in elders. These causes of falls are preventable. Often the initial evaluation of the environment by prehospital providers is the only source of information available to physicians and other health care providers to trigger prevention measures.

Motor vehicle crashes.   Impaired driving skills as a result of worsening vision, hearing, reaction time, and ability to rotate the neck as well as increased incidence of syncope in elders are predisposing factors for involvement in motor vehicle crashes (MVCs). Elder pedestrians are also more likely to be struck by motor vehicles in part as a result of diminished reaction and response times. Elders are more vulnerable to musculoskeletal trauma in MVCs.

RETURNING TO THE CASE

The patient has suffered a fall. The initial and focused assessments suggest that the patient has injuries of the head, neck, and right leg. The patient may have had a loss of consciousness. The HR of 45 is concerning. You place the patient on a monitor, start an IV of normal saline at TKO, administer oxygen by mask, and contact medical control. You prepare 1 mg of atropine for intravenous administration. Medical control asks you to hold

(continued)

off for now, because the blood pressure is adequate and the patient is stable.

The position of the right leg suggests a right hip fracture. You prepare the patient for transport by immobilizing the cervical spine, and brace the right leg with pillows and other supports to avoid unnecessary movement during transport. You obtain the patient's medical history and list of current medications from the nursing home staff. This information is vital to the emergency department staff when they evaluate this patient. It is easy to focus on the obvious hip injury, forgetting that this patient fell for reasons that must be discovered (a slip, syncope, weakness, vertigo?), sustaining head and neck injury as well. Always keep the whole patient and the whole injury in mind while treating the patient to avoid missing another injury or an acute underlying medical problem. If the patient is in severe pain, you may administer small doses of parenteral morphine (1–2 mg IV) according to regional protocols.

INITIAL EVALUATION AND TREATMENT CONSIDERATIONS IN ELDER MUSCULOSKELETAL TRAUMA

Although elder people are subject to the same mechanisms of injury as the rest of the population, their response to injury is unique. Traditional trauma care protocols, which commonly improve outcome in young patients, may not be adaptable for elders. The declining overall health and the reduced physiological reserve of elders are factors associated with poor outcome from trauma. Prehospital and in-hospital care deficiencies tend to compound the morbidity and mortality suffered by elders from multiple trauma.

The principles for approaching the multiply injured patient in the prehospital setting remain the same for the elder population. Priority must be given to the components of the initial assessment (ABCs). Initially, the airway must be opened and secured using a manual airway maneuver, oropharyngeal and nasopharyngeal airway adjuncts, or by endotracheal intubation, and in cases in which these measures fail, a surgical cricothyrotomy. Concurrent with the maintenance of the airway, stabilization and immobilization of the cervical spine must be a priority in order to prevent spinal cord injury in the presence of an occult vertebral fracture or ligamentous neck injury compromising the integrity of the spinal column. Initially, the immobilization of the cervical spine may be accomplished by manually holding the head in the neutral anatomical position. This position must be maintained during movement, transport, and performance of procedures such as intubation. This is best accomplished by a properly applied hard cervical collar, placing the patient on a hard board and securing the patient's head to the board with rigid foam lateral support material, and tape. In the elder patient with arthritis of the neck, in which the neck is stiffly held in flexion, or in patients with severe thoracic kyphosis secondary to osteoporosis, this process may pose a significant challenge. Proper immobilization in this setting may require additional padding under the head to provide support.

After the airway is secured and cervical spine immobilized, proper ventilation must be assured. If the patient has sufficient ventilation rate and effort, supplemental oxygen by non-rebreather mask at 10–15 l/min must be administered. If there is question about prior chronic obstructive pulmonary disease (COPD) history with carbon dioxide retention, supplemental oxygen should still be given, but careful monitoring of the patient for signs and symptoms of respiratory depression should ensue. If ventilation rate and effort are insufficient, assistance should be provided with bag–valve mask ventilation with high flow oxygen. Concurrently, other causes of ventilation compromise, such as tension pneumothorax or open pneumothorax, should be addressed immediately (see Chapter 13).

Adequate circulation of blood should be maintained in the patient. If there is massive hemorrhage, it should be controlled with local pressure. Pericardial tamponade and shock should be treated immediately. Patients should be resuscitated with intravenous crystalloid fluid (0.9 percent normal saline or lactated ringer's solution) through large-bore intravenous catheters. Pneumatic anti-shock garment (PASG, or military anti-shock trousers, MAST) use is controversial in multiple trauma. Although its use may be detrimental in penetrating thoracoabdominal trauma, PASG may have a role in fracture stabilization, particularly stabilization of pelvic fractures. Local protocols should dictate the use of PASG in the prehospital setting.

Only when the initial assessment of the injured elder patient is complete can the focused assessment of musculoskeletal trauma begin. However, the possible role of musculoskeletal trauma in the immediate morbidity and mortality of the trauma patient should not be underestimated. Elder patients who have a poor physiological reserve may succumb to shock from blood loss as the result of a pelvic fracture or go into shock from femur and other long-bone fractures. Therefore, proper immobilization and, where protocols dictate, proper and prompt application of appropriate traction splints (such as the Hare traction splint for mid-shaft femur fractures) may be life saving for elder patients involved in multiple trauma.

Core body temperature should not be allowed to drop. The patient should be removed from the cold environment as soon as possible. All clothing should be removed and the patient covered with blankets. If the patient's head is uninjured, cover the head if possible to protect against heat loss. The ambulance should be preheated whenever possible prior to response.

COMMONLY SEEN FRACTURES IN ELDERS

Proximal Femur (Hip)

The incidence of hip fractures starts rising after the age of 50. Hip fractures are more common among white females and least frequent in the African-American population. Institutionalized patients are at a high risk for hip fractures. Alzheimer's disease and previous fractures (particularly previous hip fracture) are predisposing factors for hip fractures.

The type of fracture determines the clinical presentation. Patients who have sustained nondisplaced hip fractures may have little pain and be able to ambulate. Displaced fractures of the hip are more symptomatic, presenting with pain, particularly associated with motion, inability to bear weight or ambulate. These fractures classically present with a shortened and externally rotated lower extremity.

Fractures of the hip can be classified as femoral neck, intertrochanteric, greater trochanter, lesser trochanter, and subtrochanteric fractures.

Initial assessment should include the initial survey for immediately life-threatening complications, followed by a thorough focused assessment. Examination of the lower extremity should include notation of the position of the patient and lower extremity. The extremity should be exposed and any swelling, tenderness, abrasions, or lacerations near the injury and deformity should be noted. Pulses in the femoral, popliteal, posterior tibial, and dorsalis pedis arteries should be recorded. Notation should be made of the color and temperature of the extremity. Sensation (assessed by touching the skin lightly or gently with a sharp object) and motor function should be assessed. In addition to the lower extremity, examination of the pelvis and back should be conducted.

The lower extremity should be immobilized in the position found, unless the distal circulation is compromised (absent or diminished pulses compared to the contralateral side, causing a cyanotic or cool extremity). If there is compromise of the distal circulation, any angulation of the lower extremity may be corrected by contacting medical control for definitive instruction. Usually applying gentle traction and positioning the extremity in neutral anatomical position is sufficient. If the patient's injury is isolated to the extremity, the use of narcotic analgesics should be considered with the direction of the on-line physician.

Vertebra

Fractures of the vertebral body are the most common fractures in elders. Vertebral body fractures in elders may result from minor trauma involving little energy transfer. Several factors associated with the changes in the spinal column that are seen with progressive age make some of the vertebral injuries seen in the elder spine unique. Some changes in the spine associated with aging are:

Progressive decrease in spinal mobility

Reduction in the diameter of the spinal canal

Decrease in bone density

Progressive degeneration of the intervertebral disc

These changes in the aging spine reduce the ability of the backbone to resist compressive forces and increase the likelihood of spinal cord injury, even with minor fractures.

Several common mechanisms of vertebral fractures have been identified. Some common injury mechanisms are hyperextension and distraction, resulting in occipitocervical dislocation; flexion and compression, resulting in a burst fracture of the first cervical vertebral body (Jefferson fracture); hyperextension, resulting in a fracture of the second vertebra (Hangman's fracture); and flexion injury, resulting in fracture dislocations and flexion and distraction injury from seatbelt (lap only), resulting in fracture dislocation in the thoracolumbar spine. Injuries with these common mechanisms should prompt the prehospital health care provider to have a high index of suspicion for vertebral and spinal cord injury.

Head and facial injury in elders should alert the prehospital health care provider to the possibility of a cervical spine injury. Altered mental status, use of intoxicants (alcohol or drugs), and concomitant injuries may confound the findings associated with spinal injury. Therefore, spinal immobilization should be the rule, not the exception, in elders with any possibility of trauma to the cervical spine.

The full range of complete and incomplete spinal cord lesions may be seen in association with vertebral fractures in elders. Some spinal cord injuries may even be seen with no vertebral injury. Central cord syndrome, characterized by quadriparesis (weakness of all four extremities) involving the upper extremities greater than the lower extremities, usually resulting from cervical hyperextension, is the most common partial cord lesion seen in elders. However, Brown–Sequard syndrome, a hemisection of the spinal cord, is rarely seen in elders and is usually a result of direct penetrating trauma to the spinal cord, such as a gunshot wound or knife injury.

The absence of sensation and muscle function below the site of injury usually indicates a complete spinal cord lesion. The distinction between complete and partial cord lesions does not need to be made in the prehospital setting, and any abnormal neurological finding should be treated as a complete cord lesion, with meticulous spinal immobilization and careful handling of the patient during all phases of prehospital care.

Distal Radius

The distal radius is a common site of fractures. Elders have an increased incidence of fractures to the distal radius because the bone is weakened from osteoporosis and because elders sustain an increased incidence of falls that they try to break by stretching out their arms. Women, particularly women over the age of 50, are much more prone to suffer from fractures of the distal radius than are men.

The most common mechanism of injury for distal radius fractures is a fall onto an outstretched hand. The most common site of injury is the weak metaphyseal bone, resulting in a Colle's type fracture with dorsal angulation of the fractured fragments, or less commonly a Smith type fracture with volar angulation. Direct axial forces on the wrist result in comminuted intraarticular injury with impaction. Fractures in which shearing forces are prevalent are usually unstable.

While evaluating a patient with a suspected injury to the forearm, the history should include the mechanism of injury, hand dominance, occupation, and normal functional capabilities of the elder patient. The physical examination should include the proximal and distal joints with respect to the injury. Areas of swelling, tenderness, discoloration and breaks in the skin should be noted. Presence of pulses, skin color and temperature, capillary refill time, sensation, and motor function (including function of flexor and extensor tendons) should be assessed. Comparisons should be made to the uninjured extremity because deformity from prior fractures or arthritis may be present more commonly in elders.

The most common nerve injury associated with a distal radius fracture is the median nerve. Ulnar nerve damage is less commonly encountered.

The treatment of suspected forearm fracture, as with all suspected fractures, should include wound management and immobilization. It should be emphasized that exposure of the entire arm is essential for proper evaluation of forearm and wrist injuries. This must be accomplished by removing all clothing without introducing further injury, and is best accomplished by cutting the clothing. All constrictive jewelry should be removed immediately, because swelling at the site of injury and distally can progress rapidly. Various techniques for removing constrictive jewelry exist, but a detailed dissertation of those methods are beyond the scope of this book. Ice should be applied to the injured area and the injured area elevated above the heart. The extremity should be immobilized in the position found unless the distal circulation is compromised. In the case where there is a significant deformity and distal pulses are absent, the distal extremity is cold, and motor and sensory functions are impaired, prehospital fracture reduction should be considered. Medical control direction and local prehospital protocols should define the course of action. Local prehospital protocols often dictate the position of splinting.

Pelvis

Unlike young patients, traumatic pelvic fractures in elders most commonly occur with low-impact trauma, such as falls from standing. Trauma to the pelvis from high-energy forces are often associated with multiple injuries, including head and intraabdominal trauma.

The initial management of the patient with a traumatic pelvic injury should be directed to the initial assessment and treatment of the airway, cervical spine, breathing, and circulation. The initial history should include the mechanism of injury. The focused assessment should be directed toward identifying life-threatening injuries first. Some signs of pelvic trauma include shortening and deformity of the lower extremities, ecchymoses to the buttocks and flank, crepitation, and instability of the pelvic ring with distraction of the iliac wings on manual compression. The perineum and male urethral meatus should be inspected for blood and soft tissue trauma. In order to properly assess the injured patient, exposure is critical. Care should be given to preserving the core body temperature with blankets and warming of the environment.

Initial treatment priorities include maintaining the patency of the airway along with spinal immobilization, attention to proper oxygenation and ventilation of the patient, and maintenance of adequate circulation. Supplemental oxygen and intravenous access via large-bore cannula is a priority. Fractures resulting from anteroposterior compressive forces often cause a widening of the pelvic circumference, and can result in large hematoma formation and pooling of significant blood volume. If a pelvic fracture is suspected, manipulation of the pelvis should be kept to an absolute minimum, as any motion can significantly increase blood loss. Use of military antishock trousers (MAST or PASG) may aid in acutely stabilizing the pelvic fracture and diminishing pelvic volume, therefore minimizing blood loss. Although the use of PASG in elders may be associated with complications from restriction of already poor peripheral circulation or an acute increase in peripheral vascular resistance and preload, it may slow down otherwise profuse pelvic bleeding and temporarily stabilize hemodynamic function. The use of PASG in the prehospital setting is controversial and regulated regionally.

Fracture Prevention in Elders

Controlling the factors that predispose elders to sustain fractures is the mainstay of fracture prevention. Control of osteoporosis by diet and pharmacology may reduce fracture rate and severity in elders. Modifying the rate of falls in elders is also an important factor in reducing musculoskeletal injuries. Control of factors that influence falls, such as worsening eyesight and unmanaged medical problems, decreases the number of falls and reduces injury rates. Reduction of environmental factors that influence falls in elders is also one area that may have an impact on reduction of falls and fall-related injury in elders. Prehospital health care professionals, including EMTs, paramedics, visiting nurses, and other home health personnel, have the advantage of firsthand viewing the environment in which elders live. These personnel may be instrumental in influencing change by direct on-site intervention through hospital or health maintenance organization (HMO) sponsored programs, or by raising awareness among health care providers concerning existing risk factors.

CASE OUTCOME

In the emergency department, x-rays reveal that the patient has a right-sided intertrochanteric fracture of the hip. Cervical spine films are negative, as is the head CT. Cardiac work-up shows that the patient has sick sinus syndrome with bradycardia and prolonged pauses. The cardiologist believes that the dysrrhythmia caused the patient to experience syncope and fall. He gets a pacemaker and is taken to the operating room for total hip replacement. He is discharged to a rehabilitation facility on the eighth hospital day and is recovering well.

REVIEW QUESTIONS

1. The most important risk factor for skeletal fractures in elders is
   a. decreased reaction time
   b. chronic illness
   c. multiple medications
   d. osteoporosis

2. Osteoporosis is commonly associated with all of the following fractures in elders *except*
   a. femur fractures
   b. hip fractures
   c. vertebral body fractures
   d. distal radius fractures

3. What percentage of elder patients fall in a given year?
   a. 10 percent
   b. 33 percent
   c. 50 percent
   d. 75 percent

4. All of the following are associated with falls in elders *except*
   a. underlying medical conditions
   b. electrical cords
   c. kyphosis of the thoracic spine
   d. antidepressant use

5. The use of the pneumatic anti-shock garment (PASG) in elder musculoskeletal trauma is
   a. controversial and frequently regulated by regional protocols
   b. is always indicated with suspected pelvic fractures
   c. is indicated for stabilization of long-bone fractures on long transports
   d. cannot cause congestive heart failure if the patient is already in shock

6. All of the following are reasons that elders are more likely than younger people to have spinal cord injury as a result of trauma *except*
   a. decrease in spinal mobility
   b. reduction in diameter of the spinal canal
   c. difficulty in immobilizing the cervical spine in patients with kyphosis
   d. decrease in bone density

7. All of the following are true about the prehospital management of suspected forearm fractures *except*
   a. the extremity should be immobilized in the position found, even if pulses are absent
   b. expose the entire injured extremity
   c. remove all constrictive jewelry
   d. application of ice

8. If a fracture of the pelvis is suspected in an elder patient
   a. only minimal bleeding should be expected
   b. movement of the pelvis should be kept to an absolute minimum
   c. abdominal injury is unlikely
   d. use of the PASG should be avoided

9. The prehospital provider can be effective in preventing fractures in elders by
   a. administering drugs to treat osteoporosis
   b. identifying environmental factors that may cause elders to fall
   c. encouraging patients to make dietary change to reduce osteoporosis
   d. all of the above

SUGGESTED READING

Knoop, K. J., L. B. Stack, and A. B. Storrow, eds. 1997. *Atlas of emergency medicine.* New York: McGraw-Hill.

Koval, K. J. and J. D. Zuckerman, eds. 1998. *Fractures in the elderly.* Philadelphia: Lippincott–Raven.

Rosen, P. and R. Barkin, eds. 1998. *Emergency medicine concepts and clinical practice,* 4th ed. St Louis: Mosby Year Book.

SECTION IV

Pharmacology

Chapter 16 Pharmacology for Prehospital Emergency Care

16

Pharmacology for Prehospital Emergency Care

Lawrence Proano, MD

OBJECTIVES

By the end of this chapter, the prehospital health care provider should be able to:

1 Discuss the physiologic differences in elder patients that affect pharmacologic treatment.

2 Identify the differences in pharmacokinetics of medications administered to elder patients.

3 Discuss the mechanism of action, indications, contraindications, adverse reactions, dosages, and drug–drug interactions for medications commonly given to elders in the prehospital setting.

4 Recognize special considerations to be aware of when administering medications to elders in the prehospital setting.

Demographic studies show that the proportion of elders in the U.S. population is increasing. Advancing age brings with it a higher incidence of disease, which increases the likelihood that an individual is taking one or more medications. In addition, elder people have an increased incidence and need for transport to hospitals for medical care. During these transports, multiple medications are frequently administered. To provide the best care for elders in the prehospital setting, providers must be aware of the special physiologic and pharmacologic issues that relate to this population.

There are several natural physiologic changes that occur with aging that have an impact on pharmacologic management of elder patients. These include

A decrease in the percentage of lean muscle mass.
An increase in the percentage of fat.
A decrease in serum protein and albumin concentration.
A decrease in total body water.

These physiologic changes, in turn, result in alterations in the pharmacokinetics of drugs in older individuals. These pharmacokinetic changes include

Decreased clearance of drugs as the result of a decline in renal function.
Altered distribution of drugs in serum and tissues.
Decreased enzymatic breakdown of drugs as a result of a decline in hepatic blood flow and decreased enzymatic activity.

As a result of these anatomic and physiologic changes, the clinical effects of most drugs are enhanced at a given concentration when administered to an older person. Any toxicity or side effect associated with a given drug is magnified in elders. Medications should be administered in elders for narrowly defined indications and at the lowest possible effective dose.

Elders, by virtue of having a greater number of chronic illnesses or conditions compared to younger patients, are often taking several medications. These medications can interact with each other, with medications administered by prehospital providers, or can cause clinical symptoms by themselves. For this reason, prehospital providers should be familiar with the medications that they administer in the emergency setting, and also have a basic understanding and awareness of the numerous medications that elder patients may take on a regular basis.

Medication actions and interactions are common causes of calls for emergency care in elders. Many of the complaints that elder patients present with are often found to be directly or indirectly related to medications they take. These complaints often do not have an obvious pharmacologic basis. For example, a patient who presents with a fall may have sustained the injury from having an episode of low blood pressure, which may have been precipitated by a tranquilizer or an antihypertensive medication. It is therefore important for prehospital providers to be cognizant of the association that medications may have with commonly presenting symptoms and complaints in elder patients.

In addition to awareness of pharmacologic principles in elders, prehospital providers can further assist in the complete and accurate assessment of the elder patient by bringing a complete list of the patient's medications to the emergency department. A complete list or bag of medications can often be the most important element of the history in diagnosing a patient's problem, for both the prehospital provider and the physician. If this critical information is left at the scene, the emergency physician may have no way of obtaining it, and the patient's care may be compromised.

This chapter covers the areas most relevant and important to the care of elder patients in the prehospital setting. In particular, it focuses on the special precautions and considerations in treating this population.

The medications covered here comprise the majority of drugs used in prehospital care of elder patients. These include a number of subcategories such as antiarrythmics, sympathomimetics, parasympatholytics, vasodilators, and cardiac glycosides.

ANTIARRHYTHMIC AGENTS

Lidocaine

Description. Lidocaine is an amide-class anesthetic with well-described antiarrythmic properties.

Mechanism of action. Lidocaine suppresses ventricular irritability by decreasing the natural automaticity and depolarization of the ventricles. In therapeutic concentrations, it has little effect on atrial tissues or on myocardial contractility. Most often, ventricular irritability occurs in the setting of acute myocardial infarction. In the face of acute myocardial ischemia, the threshold for ventricular fibrillation is reduced. Lidocaine has been shown to reduce the incidence of ventricular fibrillation. It also reduces the incidence and frequency of premature ventricular contractions (PVCs), which have been implicated as a trigger for ventricular fibrillation. Certain patterns of premature contractions are more likely than others to lead to ventricular arrythmias. These include

PVCs originating from more than one focus.

PVCs that occur in runs of two or more in a row.

PVCs that occur in certain periods of higher risk in the cardiac cycle, specifically the T wave of the preceding beat (R on T phenomenon).

Contraindications.   Lidocaine is contraindicated in patients with a hypersensitivity to the amide class of anesthetics.

Adverse reactions

Cardiovascular—Bradycardia, hypotension, cardiovascular collapse.

Allergic—Urticaria, anaphylactic reaction.

Central Nervous System (CNS)—Adverse CNS effects are variable and relate to depressive or stimulatory effects. There is a wide range of clinical effects seen, including agitation, euphoria, confusion, dizziness, numbness, tingling, tremors, twitching, seizures. There may also be drowsiness, unconsciousness, and respiratory arrest.

Indications.   Lidocaine is indicated if there is evidence of ventricular irritability, ventricular tachycardia, or ventricular fibrillation. It should also be used after the termination of such arrythmias to prevent recurrences. However, prophylactic use of lidocaine in patients with acute myocardial infarction is not recommended, as mortality has not shown to be reduced in the prehospital setting.

Dosage.   An initial dose of 1.0–1.5 mg/kg is recommended for patients with ventricular arrythmias. After the initial bolus, repeat boluses of 0.5–0.75 mg/kg may be repeated every 5–10 min to a maximum dose of 3.0 mg/kg. Because of its short half-life, lidocaine requires an infusion to maintain a therapeutic serum concentration. The maintenance infusion rate is 1–4 mg/min.

In patients in full cardiac arrest, there is poor circulation and blood flow, even with excellent cardiopulmonary resuscitation (CPR). As a result, only bolus administration of lidocaine is recommended for these patients. Once spontaneous rhythm is restored, an intravenous infusion of 1–4 mg/min may be started.

Drug–drug interactions.   Lidocaine should be used with caution when administered with other cardioactive drugs such as procainamide, quinidine, and beta-blockers. Such combinations of drugs may result in clinically toxic effects and myocardial depression.

Special considerations in elders.   Elder patients have a smaller volume of distribution, and the *maintenance* dose should be reduced to allow for this, although the loading dose would remain unchanged. A maintenance dose of 1–2 mg/min would be a reasonable place to start in an elder patient. Lidocaine is metabolized by the liver, and any condition resulting in impaired hepatic blood flow (acute myocardial infarction, congestive heart failure) should similarly prompt a reduction in the maintenance rate.

Procainamide

Description. Procainamide is an ester-class anesthetic with well-described ventricular antiarrythmic properties.

Mechanism of action. Procainamide suppresses ventricular automaticity, and may be effective in cases refractory to therapy with lidocaine. Like lidocaine, procainamide suppresses phase 4 diastolic depolarization. However, procainamide also prolongs repolarization and slows intraventricular conduction to a much greater degree than lidocaine.

Contraindications. Procainamide is contraindicated in patients with a hypersensitivity to the ester class of anesthetics, or to patients with disturbances of the conduction system.

Adverse reactions
Cardiovascular—Bradycardia, hypotension, cardiovascular collapse.
Allergic—Urticaria, anaphylactic reaction.
CNS—Adverse CNS effects are variable and relate to depression or stimulatory effects. Like lidocaine, there is a wide range of clinical effects seen, including agitation, euphoria, confusion, dizziness, numbness, tingling, tremors, twitching, and seizures. There may also be drowsiness, unconsciousness, and respiratory arrest.

Indications. Procainamide is indicated if there is evidence of ventricular irritability, ventricular tachycardia, or ventricular fibrillation, particularly in cases where lidocaine has proved ineffective. Because of its effect on atrioventricular (AV) conduction, procainamide is also useful in converting supraventricular and reentrant tachyarrhythmias.

Dosage. The intravenous dose of procainamide to suppress ventricular ectopy is 20 mg/min until ectopy is terminated or a maximum dose of 17 mg/kg is infused. The infusion should also be discontinued if the patient develops hypotension or if the QRS complex widens by more than 50 percent of its original width. If the elder patient is known to have cardiac or renal dysfunction, the total dose should be reduced to 12 mg/kg. Because of its short half-life, procainamide requires an infusion to maintain a therapeutic serum concentration. The maintenance dose is 1–4 mg/min with the lower rate recommended for elder patients.

Drug–drug interactions. Procainamide should be used with caution when administered to patients already taking procainamide, and with other cardioactive drugs such as quinidine and beta blockers. Procainamide should also be used cautiously with drugs that prolong the QRS complex, including amiodarone and sotalol. Such combinations of drugs may result in clinically toxic effects and myocardial depression.

Special considerations in elders. Procainamide has potent vasodilatory and negative inotropic effects. Elder patients, particularly if they are dehydrated, in congestive heart failure (CHF) or renal failure are more susceptible to such effects, and allowances in the dose and maintenance infusion should be made in these situations.

Amiodarone

Description. Amiodarone is an antiarrhythmic effective against ventricular arrhythmias.

Mechanism of action. Amiodarone suppresses arrhythmias by prolonging the refractory period in cardiac muscle cells. Amiodarone also inhibits both alpha and beta adrenergic receptors, causing relaxation of vascular smooth muscle and decreasing peripheral vascular resistance (reduces afterload). Because amiodarone can prolong the refractory period in all cardiac tissues, it can also cause sinus bradycardia, sinus arrest, or heart block.

Contraindications. Amiodarone is contraindicated in sinus bradycardia and second- or third-degree heart block. It is also contraindicated in patients with known hypersensitivity to the drug.

Adverse reactions. Amiodarone may cause vasodilation and hypotension, and it may also have negative inotropic effects. Amiodarone may also cause prolongation of the QT interval, so it should not be given simultaneously with other drugs that prolong the QT interval, such as procainamide. Amiodarone has a long half-life, and should be used cautiously in patients with renal failure.

Indications. In the prehospital setting, amiodarone is indicated for the treatment of ventricular fibrillation or pulseless ventricular tachycardia that is unresponsive to defibrillation. It can also be used in the treatment of wide-complex tachycardias of unclear type. It is not considered a first-line agent for ventricular arrhythmias.

Dosage. The dosage for treatment of ventricular fibrillation or pulseless ventricular tachycardia is 300 mg rapid IV push. This can be repeated as 150 mg rapid IV push in 3–5 min. For stable wide-complex tachycardias, amiodarone can be given as a rapid IV infusion of 150 mg over 10 min. This can be repeated as a second rapid IV infusion of 150 mg over 10 min. The maximum dose permissible over 24 hr is 2.2 gm IV.

Drug–drug interactions. Amiodarone should not be given concurrently with drugs that may cause prolongation of the QT interval, such as procainamide, and should be used with extreme caution in patients known to be taking such drugs.

Special considerations in elders. There is evidence that amiodarone may be useful in patients with stable ventricular tachycardia who have underlying left ventricular dysfunction (if cardioversion is unsuccessful). This situation arises most commonly in the elder population.

Elder patients are also more likely to have heart blocks, which is a contraindication to amiodarone use. Elders are also more likely to have some degree of renal dysfunction, and amiodarone should be used only with extreme caution in these patients.

Verapamil

Description. Verapamil is a calcium-channel blocker.

Mechanism of action. Verapamil inhibits slow channel activity in cardiac as well as vascular smooth muscle tissue. This serves to block the influx of sodium and calcium. As a result, verapamil produces strong negative chronotropic and inotropic effects. This serves to decrease myocardial oxygen consumption. Verapamil has been shown to slow conduction and prolong the effective refractory period in the AV node. It slows the ventricular response to atrial fibrillation and atrial flutter.

Contraindications. Verapamil is contraindicated in the setting of

Severe volume depletion or hypotension
Second- or third-degree AV block
Sick sinus syndrome
Concomitant administration of intravenous beta-blockers.

Atrial flutter or fibrillation and a known history of an accessory
   bypass tract (Wolf–Parkinson–White syndrome)
Ventricular tachycardia
Known hypersensitivity to verapamil

Adverse reactions.   Dizziness, nausea, vomiting, bradycardia, heart
block, asystole, and hypotension have all been reported with verapamil.

Indications.   Verapamil is indicated for the treatment of paroxysmal
supraventricular tachycardia (PSVT). It was formerly the drug of first
choice for emergency treatment of this rhythm, until it was supplanted
by adenosine. It terminates the most common form of PSVT by its effect of AV node inhibition. It also has some effect in slowing the ventricular response in atrial flutter and atrial fibrillation. It is now more
commonly used to treat PSVT that has not responded to adenosine.

Dosage.   For the treatment of supraventricular tachycardia, a 2.5–
5.0 mg dose is recommended in the form of an intravenous bolus
given over 2 min. If this proves ineffective, a repeat dose of 5–10 mg
can be given after about 15–30 min. A total dose of 30 mg should not
be exceeded.

Drug–drug interactions.   Verapamil is synergistic with beta-blockers.
If patients are on oral beta-blockers, or if intravenous beta-blockers are
given at the same time as verapamil, this can result in severe brady-
arrythmias, asystole, and death. In patients on digitalis, verapamil increases serum digitalis concentrations. However, unless there is
preexisting digitalis toxicity or impaired conduction through the AV
node, verapamil can be used safely.

Special considerations in elders.   Verapamil has potent electrophysiological effects. Elders are more susceptible to its side effects.
They are more likely to have preexisting left ventricular dysfunction,
placing them at greater risk for hypotension and adverse effects.

Diltiazem

Description.   Diltiazem is a calcium-channel blocker.

Mechanism of action.   Diltiazem inhibits slow channel activity in
cardiac as well as vascular smooth muscle tissue. This serves to block
the influx of sodium and calcium. Diltiazem produces strong negative chronotropic but only mild inotropic effects. It has been shown
to slow conduction and prolong the effective refractory period in the
AV node. It slows the ventricular response to atrial fibrillation and
atrial flutter.

Contraindications. Diltiazem should not be used in the setting of

Sick sinus syndrome
Second- or third-degree AV block
Severe volume depletion or hypotension
Known hypersensitivity to diltiazem
Severe left ventricular dysfunction or congestive heart failure

Adverse reactions. Dizziness, nausea, vomiting, bradycardia, heart block, asystole, and hypotension have been reported with diltiazem.

Indications. Diltiazem is effective in the treatment of PSVT. It is very effective in slowing the ventricular response in atrial flutter and atrial fibrillation.

Dosage. For the treatment of supraventricular tachycardia, a 0.25 mg/kg dose is recommended as an intravenous bolus administered over 2 min. If this proves ineffective, a repeat dose of 0.35 mg/kg can be given after about 15 min.

For ventricular rate control in the setting of atrial fibrillation or atrial flutter, an initial bolus dose of 0.25 mg/kg is given as an intravenous bolus administered over 2 min. This should be followed by a maintenance infusion at a rate of 5–15 mg/hr. The actual rate of infusion is titrated to the heart rate desired. If sufficient ventricular rate control is not achieved, a repeat bolus of 0.35 mg/kg may be given over 2 min, 15 min after the initial bolus.

Drug–drug interactions. Use caution in patients on digitalis, as diltiazem increases serum digitalis concentrations. However, unless there is preexisting digitalis toxicity or impaired conduction through the AV node, diltiazem can be used safely.

Special considerations in elders. As with verapamil, diltiazem has potent electrophysiological effects. Elders are more susceptible to its side effects. They are more likely to have preexisting left ventricular dysfunction, placing them at greater risk for hypotension and adverse effects.

Adenosine

Description. Adenosine is an endogenous purine nucleoside with antiarrythmic properties.

Mechanism of action. Adenosine slows conduction through the AV node that interrupts reentry pathways, which are a common etiology of PSVT. It has an ultrashort half-life, lasting only about 5–10 sec, before it is sequestered by red blood cells.

Contraindications.   Adenosine is contraindicated in patients with

Second- or third-degree AV block, unless there is a functioning
   artificial pacemaker
Sick sinus syndrome
Known hypersensitivity to adenosine

Adverse reactions.   Adenosine can cause a number of transient
symptoms, including facial flushing, headache, sweating, palpitations, chest pain, shortness of breath, nausea, and syncope. Because
of the extremely short half-life, treatment for these symptoms is generally not required.

Indications.   Adenosine is indicated for the treatment of PSVT, including that associated with accessory bypath tracts (Wolf–Parkinson–White syndrome), refractory to common vagal maneuvers.

Dosage.   An initial dose of 6 mg should be given as a rapid intravenous bolus, followed by a rapid 10–20 cc saline flush. If the initial
dose is unsuccessful in converting the PSVT to a normal sinus
rhythm within 1–2 min, a 12-mg dose may be administered. Another
12-mg dose may be given 1–2 min later if needed to break the PSVT.

Drug–drug interactions.   The effects of adenosine are antagonized
by methylxanthines such as caffeine and theophylline. The effects of
adenosine are potentiated by dipyridamole. Carbamazepine has been
reported to have a synergistic effect with adenosine on AV node conduction. The dose of adenosine may need to be adjusted in the presence of these medications.

Special considerations in elders.   Adenosine has a fairly good safety
profile because of its short half-life. Syncope may occur briefly when
the AV node is blocked during peak effect, which lasts only a few sec-
onds. Caution in its use in elders revolves around the same issues as
in younger patients.

MISCELLANEOUS AGENTS

Oxygen

Description.   Oxygen is a colorless and odorless gas. It is essential
for human life and a mainstay of basic supportive patient care.

Mechanism of action.   Normal inspired air contains only about 20
percent oxygen. Normally, oxygen enters the body through the lungs
and is transported by hemoglobin in red blood cells. In the capillaries, oxygen is released into the tissues, where it is used in the

metabolism of glucose for energy production. Various disease states may make oxygen less available (decreased cardiac output, pulmonary conditions, shunting). In this setting, supplemental oxygen administered by health care providers helps correct these deficiencies.

Contraindications. There are no contraindications for oxygen in the prehospital setting. There is a relative contraindication to giving too much oxygen to patients who have chronic obstructive pulmonary disease (COPD) who are CO_2 retainers. However, it is important to remember the dictum that oxygen should never be withheld from a hypoxic patient because of fear of possible respiratory depression.

Adverse reactions. There are no adverse reactions to oxygen for short-term course such as in the prehospital setting.

Indications. Oxygen is indicated for patients who have suspected or actual hypoxia. It is given to patients with most urgent or emergent conditions as general supportive care. In particular, it is given to patients with chest pain and respiratory difficulty. Oxygen is also given to patients with suspected carbon monoxide poisoning.

Dosage. Oxygen is given by nasal cannula, face mask, bag–valve mask, or via endotracheal tube. The dosage is measured in the form of inspired percent, or in liters per minute of flow. For conditions of minor or intermediate severity, a flow rate of 2–6 l/min by nasal cannula is usually given. For more severe conditions or greater degrees of hypoxia, or in cases of suspected carbon monoxide poisoning, oxygen is administered by non-rebreather face mask, with a flow rate of 10–15 l/min. In the case of cardiac arrest, oxygen is administered by bag–valve mask or endotracheal tube at an inspired concentration of 100 percent at 10–15 l/min.

Drug–drug interactions. There are no interactions between oxygen and any prescription or over-the-counter medications.

Special considerations in elders. The main consideration in elder as well as younger patients is to assure that there is adequate oxygenation. Without this prerequisite, all other interventions may prove futile.

Sodium Bicarbonate

Description. Sodium bicarbonate is a salt solution that buffers metabolic acidosis.

Mechanism of action. Sodium bicarbonate provides bicarbonate molecules to buffer excess hydrogen ions produced in the setting of tissue hypoperfusion. Multiple controlled studies have shown that the acidosis that results from poor tissue perfusion does not affect the ability to defibrillate, as formerly thought, nor does it decrease the ability to restore circulation with a spontaneous cardiac rhythm. There is no evidence that it improves survival rates following cardiac arrest. In addition, the use of bicarbonate has the potential to induce alkalemia, hyperosmolality, hypernatremia, and paradoxical intracellular acidosis.

Contraindications.   There are no absolute contraindications to the use of sodium bicarbonate.

Adverse reactions.   There are no overtly recognizable adverse reactions seen with bicarbonate administration. However, it may produce deleterious effects at the cellular level that do not aid in improving the emergent condition for which it is given.

Indications.   Current concepts of acid-base physiology lead to very limited indications for sodium bicarbonate. These are

As a last resort in the management of cardiac arrest.
In the treatment of tricyclic antidepressant overdose to correct cardiac arrythmias and aid in renal excretion.
In the treatment of phenobarbital overdose, to aid in renal excretion.
In the treatment of hyperkalemia.
In the treatment of severe acidosis that is not rapidly correctable by other means.

Dosage.   The initial dose of sodium bicarbonate is 1 mEq/kg of body weight by intravenous bolus. This is followed by subsequent doses of 0.5 mEq/kg every 10 min. If bicarbonate is given, its effect should be monitored by blood gas analysis.

Drug–drug interactions.   Catecholamines such as epinephrine and dopamine are inactivated by sodium bicarbonate. Therefore, before these drugs are given concurrently, the intravenous line should be flushed or a different access line should be used. It should also not be given in close conjunction with calcium chloride, as it forms a precipitate in the intravenous line.

Special considerations in elders.   Elders are the most likely victims of cardiac arrest. It is important for clinicians to be aware of the limitations and potential dangers of this agent. It is important to bear in mind that 1 ampule of sodium bicarbonate contains as much sodium as 1 l of normal saline, and if used inappropriately, may cause fluid retention and CHF in elder patients.

Atropine

Description. Atropine is a parasympatholytic agent with anticholinergic effects.

Mechanism of action. Atropine inhibits the parasympathetic system by blocking acetylcholine receptors. Its inhibitory effect on the vagus nerve results in an increase in the heart rate. It has positive chronotropic effects but no inotropic effects. It improves sinus node automaticity and AV node conduction. In the setting of asystole, it may have a beneficial effect, as there is some evidence that asystole may be accompanied by a dramatic increase in parasympathetic tone.

Contraindications. Atropine has no absolute contraindications, but it should be used judiciously, especially in patients with potential myocardial ischemia, in whom tachycardia may have deleterious effects. Although it is useful in the treatment of first-degree AV block and Mobitz type I AV block, it has been reported to be harmful in some patients who have high-degree AV block (Mobitz type II and third-degree AV block).

Adverse reactions. Excessive doses may cause tachycardia, blurred vision, mydriasis (pupilary dilatation), dry mouth, drowsiness, dizziness, and confusion.

Indications. Atropine is indicated for hemodynamically significant bradycardias. This is generally defined as a heart rate less than 50 beats per minute (bpm), or a heart rate that is in the normal range but accompanied by hypotension, chest pain, CHF, or confusion. It may be useful in the treatment of patients with excessive vagal tone causing sinus or nodal bradycardia. This is often seen in the setting of acute myocardial infarction, particularly in the inferior distribution. Atropine should also be considered in the management of symptomatic bradycardias as a result of organophosphate poisoning.

Dosage. The usual dose of atropine is 0.5 mg administered intravenously. This may be repeated at 5-min intervals until the desired effect is reached or until a maximum total dose of 0.04 mg/kg is reached (2–3 mg for most adults). In treating asystole in cardiac arrest, the initial dose is 1.0 mg administered intravenously. If intravenous access is unavailable, it can also be given via an endotracheal tube. In this case, the dose is 1–2 mg diluted in 5–10 cc of normal saline.

Drug–drug interactions. There are no significant interactions with other drugs.

Special considerations in elders. Prehospital providers should be familiar with atropine and its use, as it is frequently indicated in elder patients.

Nitroglycerin

Description. Nitroglycerin is a simple chemical in the organic nitrate family with a potent smooth muscle relaxant effect.

Mechanism of action. Nitroglycerin relaxes smooth muscle in both arteries and veins by stimulating specific receptors. Nitroglycerin dilates the coronary arteries and increases coronary blood flow to ischemic areas of the heart. This reduces the chest pain felt with angina pectoris, usually within 1–3 min. Through its vasodilatation, nitroglycerin reduces preload, which in turn decreases cardiac work and oxygen consumption. In patients with CHF, nitroglycerin reduces left ventricular filling pressure as well as total systemic vascular resistance, which often improves the clinical picture.

Contraindications. Nitroglycerin is contraindicated in the presence of hypotension.

Adverse reactions. Common side effects include facial flushing, headache, hypotension, nausea, vomiting, and bradycardia. Most elder patients on long-term nitrogycerine therapy develop tolerance to these side effects.

Indications. Nitroglycerin is indicated for the treatment of acute angina pectoris. It is also indicated for patients with acute CHF as long as they are not hypotensive.

Dosage. The usual dose is one (0.4 mg) tablet sublingually. A similar dosage can be given orally as a spray. This is repeated at 5-min intervals to a maximum dose of three tablets.

Drug–drug interactions. Nitroglycerin's hypotensive effects can be exacerbated in the setting of volume depletion or when used in conjunction with beta blockers.

Special considerations in elders. Elders are certainly the most likely candidates to require the use of nitroglycerin. They are also the most susceptible to its side effects, including hypotension. Elder patients are often volume depleted and may be taking prescribed beta-blockers. Hypotension can be serious in this population if it is severe enough to impair tissue perfusion and cause or worsen myocardial ischemia. Elder patients with preexisting aortic valve stenosis may have syncope after receiving nitroglycerin. Caution should be used in elders, and vital signs should be monitored closely. It is safe to use nitroglycerin in elder patients who have had angioplasty, coronary stents, and coronary artery bypass graft procedures.

Furosemide

Description.   Furosemide is a potent loop diuretic, useful in the treatment of CHF.

Mechanism of action.   Furosemide acts by inhibiting reabsorption of sodium and chloride in the ascending loop of Henle in the kidney. In addition, it has vasodilating effects that result in reduced venous return to the heart, which reduces preload. The diuretic effect begins within about 10 min of administration, but the vasodilating effects begin even sooner. This biphasic effect makes it extemely useful in the treatment of CHF.

Contraindications.   Administration is contraindicated in patients who have a known hypersensitivity to furosemide or sulfonamides.

Adverse reactions.   With overly aggressive diuresis, hypotension, hypokalemia, hyponatremia, and hypochloremia are seen. These are not generally seen in the prehospital setting, but inappropriate use of furosemide may cause these problems later in the hospital setting.

Indications.   Furosemide is the drug of choice in the initial treatment of CHF.

Dosage.   The initial dose of furosemide is 20–40 mg. It is given by slow intravenous push over 1–2 min. Higher initial doses may be necessary in elder patients who are already taking large daily doses of furosemide. Follow local protocols or contact on-line medical control as necessary.

Drug–drug interactions.   Use caution when administering furosemide and nitroglycerin together in the elder patient, as they are synergistic in preload reduction.

Special considerations in elders.   Elders often present with acute respiratory distress. This can be caused by CHF, pneumonia, or an exacerbation of asthma or COPD. The only one of these for which furosemide is indicated is CHF. The distinction between these conditions in elders can often be difficult, especially in the prehospital setting. Furosemide can be harmful if given to an elder patient who is dehydrated and has pneumonia, and whose pulmonary rales were mistaken for CHF. Therefore, it is important for prehospital providers to develop a strong clinical acumen to distinguish these entities.

Epinephrine

Description.   Epinephrine is a natural catecholamine. It has potent alpha- and beta-adrenergic activity.

Mechanism of action.   Epinephrine's adrenergic stimulation results in increased heart rate, blood pressure, systemic vascular resistance, coronary blood flow, cardiac contractile force, and automaticity. In the setting of asystole, it can restore spontaneous cardiac activity. In addition, epinephrine causes bronchodilation from its beta-adrenergic effect. Finally, epinephrine also counteracts the effects of anaphylaxis, including the bronchoconstriction that accompanies it.

Contraindications.   Epinephrine should be used with caution or not at all in patients with cardiovascular disease or high blood pressure.

Adverse reactions.   Epinephrine can cause cardiac ischemia, heart palpitations, agitation, headache, dizziness, nausea, and vomiting.

Indications.   Epinephrine is indicated for the treatment of

Cardiac arrest with asystole, ventricular fibrillation, ventricular tachycardia, or pulseless electrical activity.
Acute bronochspasm associated with asthma and severe COPD.
Acute severe anaphylaxis.

Dosage.   The standard common dose of epinephrine in cardiac arrest is 1.0–1.5 mg of a 1:10,000 solution intravenously. This dosage is doubled if administered via an endotracheal tube. This is repeated every 3–5 min if necessary. There is some experimental evidence to suggest that higher dose epinephrine may be successful in the cardiac arrest setting, but it is currently inconclusive. In the absence of a functioning intravenous line, epinephrine may be given via an endotracheal tube (2.0–2.5 mg diluted in 10 ml normal saline). For the treatment of severe anaphylaxis, the initial dose should be 0.3–0.5 mg intravenously. This is repeated as often as every 5 min as needed.

Drug–drug interactions.   Catecholamines are inactivated by alkaline solutions, so epinephrine should not be given at the same time as sodium bicarbonate. Epinephrine can exacerbate ventricular irritability in elder patients who are on digitalis.

Special considerations in elders.   The main concern with using epinephrine in elders is the potential for adverse effects in those patients who have underlying cardiovascular disease. Epinephrine may cause cardiac ischemia, angina, and increased myocardial oxygen demand. Nevertheless, it should not be withheld when there is a clear indication for its use, as it can be life saving.

Morphine

Description. Morphine is a narcotic analgesic.

Mechanism of action. Morphine is a narcotic agent that acts on opiate receptors in the brain. In so doing, it produces a number of central and peripheral effects. Centrally, it provides potent analgesic effects. It has powerful CNS depressant effects that result in dose-related respiratory depression. Peripherally, it produces increased venous capacitance, which decreases systemic vascular resistance. This decreased systemic vascular resistance serves to lessen myocardial oxygen demand.

Contraindications. Morphine is contraindicated in patients with hypersensitivity to opiates. A relative contraindication is volume depletion, which can make patients more vulnerable to hypotension.

Adverse reactions. Morphine can cause nausea, vomiting, meiosis (constricted pupils), blurred vision, CNS depression, and respiratory depression.

Indications. Morphine is indicated for the treatment of pain from angina pectoris and myocardial infarction. It is useful in the treatment of acute pulmonary edema. It is also occasionally used for relief of severe pain in the prehospital setting, such as burns. Refer to local protocols or contact on-line medical control for this indication.

Dosage. Morphine is administered in 1–4 mg doses intravenously. It can be repeated every 3–5 min until the desired effect is achieved while closely monitoring vital signs and watching for adverse reactions.

Drug–drug interactions. Morphine's CNS depressant effects are enhanced by other opiates, barbiturates, alcohol, sedatives, and hypnotics.

Special considerations in elders. The adverse effects of morphine, especially respiratory depression, are more pronounced in elders. Dosage reductions are recommended in this population, particularly those with known hepatic or renal impairment.

Diazepam

Description. Diazepam is an anticonvulsant and sedative in the benzodiazapine class.

Mechanism of action.   Diazepam exerts its action in the limbic system of the brain. It causes sedation and muscle relaxation, and in the setting of abnormal electrical discharge in the brain (seizures), it reduces cortical irritability.

Contraindications.   Diazepam is contraindicated in patients with known hypersensitivity to the drug. Also, diazepam should not be used in patients with acute angle closure glaucoma.

Adverse reactions.   Diazepam may cause drowsiness, ataxia, and hypotension. Excessive doses can produce respiratory depression and progressive CNS depression.

Indications.   Diazepam is indicated in the prehospital setting to treat acute seizure activity and status epilepticus.

Dosage.   To treat seizures, the usual dosage of diazepam is 5–10 mg given intravenously. It may be repeated if seizures do not resolve while monitoring respiratory status carefully. For repeat dosages, follow local protocols or contact on-line medical control.

Drug–drug interactions.   Diazepam is potentiated by alcohol and other CNS depressants. It precipitates easily, so when given in conjunction with other medications, the intravenous line should be flushed with normal saline prior to administration.

Special considerations in elders.   Dosage should be reduced in elders, especially those on prior CNS depressants.

Thiamine

Description.   Thiamine is a water-soluble vitamin, also known as vitamin B_1. It is used by the body during metabolism for the conversion of pyruvic acid to acetyl-coenzyme-A.

Mechanism of action.   Thiamine is used by the body in the metabolism of food for energy production. Thiamine, like all vitamins, is a cofactor that the body requires for metabolism but cannot produce itself. Although all tissues and cells require thiamine for energy production, the CNS is most sensitive to a lack of thiamine. If a critically low level of thiamine is reached, this can precipitate an acute confusional state known as Wernicke's syndrome. This encephalopathy is characterized by an ataxic gait, delirium, and weakness of the muscles of the eye. For these reasons, any patient with a depressed level of consciousness should receive intravenous thiamine, particularly in patients who might be alcoholic, because they are at higher risk for thiamine deficiency.

Contraindications. There are virtually no contraindications to the administration of thiamine.

Adverse reactions. Side effects are rare. Transient hypotension has been reported with intravenous administration.

Indications. Thiamine is indicated in the setting of depressed level of consciousness or coma, particularly in patients who are suspected of chronic alcohol abuse. In the setting of a diabetic patient who may also be alcoholic, thiamine should be given prior to D50W because of a theoretical concern that administering D50W prior to thiamine could cause a sudden reduction in thiamine stores and precipitate a Wernicke's encephalopathy.

Dosage. The emergency dose of thiamine is 100 mg intravenously or intramuscularly.

Drug–drug interactions. There are no significant interactions with other commonly used pharmaceuticals.

Special considerations in elders. There are no specific elder considerations for thiamine.

Naloxone

Description. Naloxone is a narcotic antagonist agent, and is used to reverse overdoses caused by drugs in the opiate class.

Mechanism of action. Naloxone works by competing for opiate receptors in the brain. This results in the competitive displacement of narcotic molecules from the opiate receptors located in the CNS. In so doing, it reverses the actions of opiate narcotic agents, including both CNS effects and respiratory depression. It is extremely effective, has a favorable side effect profile, and an excellent cost–benefit ratio.

Contraindications. There are no contraindications to the use of naloxone other than hypersensitivity to the drug, which is extremely rare.

Adverse reactions. The main adverse reactions from the use of naloxone in the prehospital setting relate to withdrawal from the reversal of narcotic depression, which can precipitate nausea, vomiting, diarrhea, diaphoresis, tachycardia, hypertension, and cardiovascular collapse. Naloxone can also precipitate severe pain crises in patients who are dependent on high-dose narcotics for pain control, such as patients with metastatic cancer.

Indications. Naloxone is indicated in the treatment of respiratory and CNS depression caused by narcotic analgesics, or as empiric treatment in coma of unknown origin.

Dosage. Generally, patients are given 1–2 mg by rapid intravenous push to treat narcotic overdoses, whether suspected or known, unintentional or intentional. In the absence of an intravenous line it may be given by endotracheal tube. Large overdoses or ingestions of certain synthetic narcotic agents such as propoxyphene may require larger or repeat doses of naloxone.

Drug–drug interactions. The only significant interaction of naloxone is with narcotic analgesics, with which it is meant to counteract.

Special considerations in elders. There are no special considerations for the use of naloxone in elder patients.

Dextrose–50 Percent in Water (D50W)

Description. Dextrose is a synonym for glucose, which is the main carbohydrate used for energy production by the body.

Mechanism of action. Fifty percent dextrose supplies glucose needed in cases of acute hypoglycemia.

Contraindications. There are no absolute contraindications to the use of 50 percent dextrose, but it should be used with caution in patients with increased intracranial pressure, because the hypertonic load may worsen cerebral edema.

Adverse reactions. The only adverse reaction to the use of dextrose is extravasation of the solution into the soft tissue. If this occurs, there can be local phlebitis or tissue necrosis.

Indications. Fifty percent dextrose is indicated in the setting of suspected or confirmed hypoglycemia, or as empiric treatment for coma of unknown origin.

Dosage. The usual dosage for the treatment of acute hypoglycemia is 50 cc of a 50 percent solution (25 g of glucose) administered intravenously.

Drug–drug interactions. There is no significant interaction with any medications.

Special considerations in elders. Confusional states and coma are common presenting symptoms in emergency calls for elder patients.

Dextrose should be considered in any elder patient who presents this way, and a history should be sought regarding possible diabetes or use of insulin or oral hypoglycemics.

REVIEW QUESTIONS

1. All of the following are physiologic changes associated with aging *except*
   a. decrease in the percentage of muscle mass
   b. decrease in serum protein content
   c. increase in percentage of body fat
   d. increase in liver clearance of drugs

2. All of the following are true about altered pharmacokinetics of drugs taken by elder persons *except*
   a. reduced effectiveness at standard dosages as a result of lowered tissue sensitivity to most drugs
   b. decreased clearance by the kidney
   c. altered distribution of drugs in the body tissues
   d. decreased ability to break down drugs

3. Elder patients receiving a lidocaine infusion may require a reduced infusion rate for all of the following reasons *except*
   a. they have a smaller volume of distribution
   b. seizure disorder
   c. acute myocardial infarction with cardiogenic shock
   d. liver disease

4. Elder patients with renal disease receiving procainamide may require a reduction in the infusion rate because
   a. they may be more susceptible to arrhythmias
   b. procainamide can worsen renal failure
   c. they may become hypotensive
   d. they may develop acute pulmonary edema

5. Bretylium should be used with caution in patients with suspected
   a. ventricular tachycardia
   b. myocardial infarction
   c. congestive heart failure
   d. digitalis toxicity

6. When administering verapamil to an elder patient, the prehospital provider should carefully monitor for
   a. atrial flutter
   b. ventricular tachycardia
   c. third-degree heart block
   d. hypotension

7. The appropriate prehospital treatment of the elder patient with known coronary artery disease who is in suspected anaphylactic shock is
   a. benadryl IV
   b. epinephrine IV
   c. dopamine IV
   d. methylprednisolone (Solumedrol) IV

8. Furosemide should be used with caution in elder patients in respiratory distress because
   a. they may develop arrhythmias
   b. they may be having a concurrent myocardial infarction
   c. they may have pneumonia or dehydration rather than congestive heart failure
   d. they may not respond to standard dosages

9. Nitroglycerin should be given with caution to elder patients with all of the following conditions *except*
   a. atrial fibrillation
   b. dehydration
   c. aortic stenosis
   d. beta blocker use

10. Diltiazem should not be used in the elder patient with all of the following conditions *except*
   a. sick sinus syndrome
   b. patients with functioning pacemakers
   c. second- or third-degree heart block
   d. congestive heart failure

SUGGESTED READING

Bledsoe, B. E., D. E. Clayden, and F. J. Papa. 1996. *Prehospital emergency pharmacology*, 4th ed. Upper Saddle River: Prentice Hall.

Hardiman, J. G., A. G. Gilman, and L. E. Limbird. 1996. *Goodman & Gilman's the pharmacological basis of therapeutics*, 9th ed. New York: MacMillan.

Judd, R. L., C. G. Warner, and M. A. Shaffer. 1986. *Geriatric Emergencies*. New York: Aspen.

SECTION V

Special Considerations

17

Elder Abuse and Neglect

Robert Partridge, MD, MPH

OBJECTIVES

By the end of this chapter, the prehospital health care provider should be able to:

1 Discuss the definition of elder abuse.
2 Recognize different types of elder abuse and neglect.
3 Discuss the obligation of the prehospital provider to report suspected elder abuse.
4 Appreciate the critical role of the prehospital provider in identifying elder abuse.

CASE

You respond to an address to evaluate an elder person who has fallen at home. On your arrival, you find an elder person on the floor in the back room of the house. A relative, the patient's niece, lives in the house and tells you that the patient fell and is unable to get up. The niece seems irritated and asks you to hurry to get her aunt to the hospital, stating "She is too much for me." The house is generally well kept except the patient's room. In it there is a bed, a chair, a walker, and a commode. The room has not been cleaned for some time, and dirty dishes and clothes litter the floor. The window shade is down at midday.

The patient is alert and oriented, and complains only of left hip pain. On initial assessment, she is in no respiratory distress with clear breath sounds, and heart rate and blood pressure are normal. Focused assessment reveals that she is thin and frail, her left hip is tender, and the left leg appears shortened and externally rotated. You also notice that she has multiple contusions on her arms, legs, and back. Some of the contusions seem to be old and others new. Her skin and clothes are soiled. The niece states that the patient has Parkinson's disease and that she falls a lot. You perform appropriate prehospital care, immobilize the patient, and prepare to transfer her to the local emergency department. On the way there, you ask the patient why she has so many bruises. She refuses to answer and begins to weep.

Aside from a left hip injury, what do you think is going on here? Is this patient a victim of abuse, or neglect, or both? What evidence do you have to support these suspicions? What should you do? Should you report your suspicions? To whom? Will your intervention make a difference for this patient?

Elder abuse is defined as "the willful infliction of injury, unreasonable confinement, intimidation or cruel punishment, with resulting physical harm or pain or mental anguish; or the willful depreciation by a caretaker of goods or services that are necessary to avoid physical harm, mental anguish or mental illness."

Elder abuse is not a new problem. It is not known whether elder abuse is more common now than in previous decades. It may seem more common now because all care providers are trained to recognize and report it. Local and state governments now have agencies that can receive and investigate reports of potential elder abuse. States also have specific laws defining elder abuse, and neglect, and criminal punishments for those who perpetrate elder abuse. Some experts suggest that elder abuse may now be more common than in previous generations because older people have a longer life expectancy and because the structure of families has changed dramatically. In the past, older people were commonly cared for by family members. Now, social factors including a larger number of single-parent families, high divorce rates with subsequent remarriages, and greater numbers of women working outside the home have placed a strain on the ability of families to care for their elders. One result of these changes may be an increase in the rate of elder abuse.

Elder abuse and neglect is now a widely recognized problem, but it receives less attention than domestic violence or child abuse. Few mechanisms exist to identify elder abuse, and as a result it frequently goes unreported. Elder abuse occurs across all socioeconomic, racial, and religious lines. Some elder persons may suffer several different types of abuse at one time. Prehospital health care providers are in a unique position to identify and report abuse and neglect in this population.

Older patients use emergency medical services at about twice the rate of other age groups and are more likely to require paramedic-accompanied transportation to hospital. The elder population (older than 65) is also the fastest growing population in the United States, making up 13 percent of the population in 1990 and expected to grow to 18 percent in 2020 and 25 percent in 2050. By the year 2020, older people will outnumber children. Even now, elders utilize emergency departments and emergency medical services more than any other age group. It is currently estimated that as many as 2.5 million elder persons are abused each year, and it is likely that over time, emergency medical services (EMS) personnel will see an increasing number of abused or neglected elder patients.

TYPES OF ABUSE

Elder mistreatment, which may be perpetuated by family members or other formal or informal caregivers, can be classified into five categories: physical abuse, psychological abuse, financial abuse, sexual abuse, and neglect.

Physical abuse is defined as the infliction of bodily harm without the elder person's consent, regardless of whether they are capable or incapable of giving consent. *Psychological abuse* is defined as the infliction of mental anguish on an elder person. *Financial* or *material abuse* is defined as the illegal or improper exploitation of an elder person's funds or resources. *Sexual abuse* includes any form of sexual exposure or contact that takes place without the older person's consent. *Neglect* is defined as the refusal or failure to fulfill a caretaking responsibility, and includes abandonment or isolation. Neglect may include denial of food, clothing, shelter, medical care, medications, or assistive devices by a person with an obligation to care for the older person. It is important to note that elder abuse and neglect can be intentional or unintentional. *Intentional abuse or neglect* refers to a conscious or deliberate attempt to mistreat an older person. *Unintentional abuse or neglect* is an unconscious or inadvertent action that harms an elder person. Unintentional abuse or neglect may occur out of ignorance, inexperience, excessive caregiver burden, or as the result of inability or lack of desire to provide appropriate care for an elder person. The definitions of abuse, physical harm, exploitation, and neglect are defined in the Elder Abuse Prevention, Identification and Treatment Act and summarized in Table 17.1.

Risk Factors for Abuse

The likelihood of elder mistreatment is increased if one or several well-known risk factors are present. Some of these are associated with the abuser, and some are associated with the victim. Any type of cognitive impairment or mental illness in the victim or a shared living arrangement between the victim and the abuser may increase the risk of abuse. Also, the frailty of older persons may also put them at risk for abuse, as they are less likely to be able to defend themselves or escape from an abusive situation.

Risk factors associated with the abuser include substance abuse or mental illness; dependence of the abuser on the elder person for financial support, housing, or other necessities (which may precipitate financial abuse); and a history of violence or other

Table 17.1. Definitions

Abuse	Willful infliction of injury, unreasonable confinement, intimidation, or cruel punishment with resulting physical harm, pain, or mental anguish; or the willful deprivation by a caretaker of goods or services that are necessary to avoid physical harm, mental anguish, or mental illness.
Physical Harm	Bodily pain, injury, impairment, or disease.
Exploitation	Illegal or improper act of a caretaker using the resources of an elder for monetary or personal benefit, profit, or gain.
Neglect	Failure of a caretaker to provide the goods or services necessary to avoid physical harm, mental anguish, or mental illness.

Adapted from Kleinschmidt, K. C. 1997. Elder abuse: A review. *Annals of Emergency Medicine* 30:463–472 (Mosby), with permission.

antisocial behavior either within or outside the family on the part of the abuser. In addition, elder people who have fewer social contacts and supports and who have had recent stressful life events (such as the death of a spouse) may also be at risk for abuse. Risk factors for elder abuse are summarized in Table 17.2. Elder abuse has not been shown to be associated with religion, education, economic background, sex, or alcohol use. Several large studies have shown some trends in the type of elder person at risk for abuse. Poor physical health is correlated with abuse. Elder persons who are unable to adequately perform activities of daily living (ADLs, such as bathing and toileting) are more likely to be neglected, especially if they have difficulty eating. Elder persons who are demented who have difficulty with ADLs are more likely to be physically abused. Neglect often affects those persons who have no one to turn to for help, who are in poor health, or who live alone. Verbal and physical abuse are more likely if the elder person lives with someone. Financial abuse more commonly affects those with no one to turn to or those who live alone.

Finally, some elder abuse may be attributed to mutually abusive relationships, or the "cycle of violence" that is sometimes seen in domestic or child abuse. As many as one-third of demented patients direct physically abusive behaviors toward their caregivers, which can result in retaliatory violence toward them from their caregivers. Violence by demented patients is increased if the patient had a poor relationship with the caregiver prior to the onset of dementia. Violence by a caregiver increases if the demented person is aggressive toward the caregiver or if they engage in disruptive behavior such as wandering, embarrassing behaviors, or verbal outbursts.

Table 17.2. **Risk Factors for Elder Mistreatment**

General
   Social isolation
   Recent stressful life event
      Death of spouse
      Financial stress

Caregiver Risk Factors
   Alcohol or drug abuse
   Mental illness
   Financial dependence on the elder person
   History of family violence or other antisocial behavior

Victim Risk Factors
   Cognitive impairment or mental illness
   Living arrangement shared with the abuser
   Poor health or functional impairment

The patient is a victim of both physical abuse and neglect. The multiple bruises of varying age, especially bruises in areas unlikely to be injured in a fall, are suggestive of physical abuse. The patient's emotional state is also suggestive of an unhealthy relationship with her niece. The deplorable condition of her living quarters is highly suggestive of neglect. On arrival in the emergency department, the patient is found to have a fractured hip, a urinary tract infection, and multiple contusions. She denies abuse to both the emergency physician and nurse, and is admitted to the hospital for repair of her fractured hip.

RECOGNITION OF ABUSE

Detection of elder abuse is often difficult. The abused elder person may be unlikely to report this abuse because of denial or shame, and health care professionals may fail to detect elder abuse either through denial or inadequate assessment. Victims of elder abuse may also feel that reporting abuse may result in loss of a caregiver and institutionalization, and this fear is well founded.

The prehospital provider is in a unique position to identify and report elder abuse and neglect. As a group, prehospital providers have regular contact with elders. As initial responders to calls for medical assistance, EMTs and paramedics often enter an elder person's dwelling as a routine part of their work, and they can identify patients whose health, social, environmental, and psychological circumstances place them at risk. It is known that paramedics are able to identify at-risk elder patients. One recent study showed that when paramedics identified an elder person who was at risk, trained geriatric assessors who followed up on this information were in agreement in 98 percent of cases.

Prehospital providers frequently assess *scene safety* under a variety of circumstances. It is important to keep scene safety in mind when responding to a call for an elder person. Is the scene in their home safe for them, and, if unsafe, is neglect or self-neglect apparent? Elder patients may simply be unaware of certain hazards, but capable of having them corrected if the hazard is brought to their attention. Other elder individuals may be incapable of taking corrective action and may be an "accident waiting to happen." If in doubt as to whether neglect or self-neglect exists, it is appropriate for the prehospital provider to contact the appropriate state or social services agency so that a more detailed home assessment can be made. Factors to be aware of are multiple. Is the dwelling adequately heated or air conditioned? Is the dwelling clean and well lighted? Do slip-and-fall hazards exist? For example, stairways should have railings, a slip-resistant surface, and no uneven sections that could cause an elder person to trip. Electrical cords, throw rugs, bathroom floors, and bathtubs without anti-slip matting are also slip-and-trip hazards. Finally, does a working telephone or emergency-alert device exist so that an elder person can summon help if needed?

Prehospital providers are uniquely positioned and capable of identifying elder abuse and neglect, and like all health professionals should maintain a high index of suspicion for this problem. Prehospital providers often see the home environment directly as well as the interaction between the elder person and his or her caregivers. Other health professionals, especially those who are hospital based (e.g., emergency department personnel), may not have the benefit of this information when making an assessment. Prehospital providers may also have the opportunity to interview the elder patient away from family members and other caregivers, so the elder person may be more inclined to offer a candid response to questions. Questions that can help to identify victims of abuse can be found in Table 17.3. These

Table 17.3. Questions Useful in Identifying Victims of Elder Abuse

Physical Abuse
  Are you afraid of anyone who cares for you or has access to your home?
  Have you been hit, slapped, or kicked by anyone?
  Have you been tied down or locked in a room?

Psychological Abuse
  Do you ever feel alone?
  Have you been threatened with punishment, deprivation, or institutionalization?
  What happens when you and your caregiver disagree?

Sexual Abuse
  Has anyone touched you without permission?

Neglect
  Is your home safe?
  Have you been left alone for long periods?
  Has anyone failed to help you care for yourself when you could not do it alone?
  Do you lack personal aids such as eyeglasses, hearing aids, or dentures?

Financial Abuse
  Is your money ever stolen or used inappropriately?
  Have you been forced to sign power of attorney, a will or another document against
    your wishes?
  Have you been forced to buy things against your wishes?
  Is your caregiver dependent on you for financial support?

Adapted from Kleinschmidt, K.C. 1997. Elder abuse: A review. *Annals of Emergency Medicine* 30:463–472 (Mosby), with permission.

questions are meant to serve as guidelines for prehospital care personnel who suspect that a patient is a victim of abuse. It is not necessary to ask each question of every elder patient encountered.

Physical exam clues to elder mistreatment can be found in Table 17.4. Many of these physical findings associated with physical and psychological abuse as well as neglect would be obvious to the prehospital provider. Complaints related to the genital area should be noted and recorded, but examination, other than that to stop profuse bleeding, should be deferred to hospital personnel. Any historical or physical findings that raise the concern of elder abuse should be reported to hospital personnel. However, all prehospital health care providers should bear in mind that these signs do not always indicate the abuse has occurred, and also that reports of abuse may not correlate with physical findings.

Of course, prehospital health care providers cannot be expected to do a detailed investigation for problems other than that for which they responded. However, they can observe the home situation and record and report problems that warrant further investigation.

Table 17.4 Physical Signs of Elder Abuse

Physical Abuse
  Bruises, wounds, or burns of various ages or patterns, well-defined
    shapes, immersion pattern
  Rope or restraint marks on wrists or ankles
  Scalp swelling or traumatic hair removal

Psychological Abuse
  Habit disorder (sucking, rocking)
  Neurotic disorders (antisocial, borderline)
  Conduct disorder

Sexual Abuse
  Genital or anal pain, itching, bruising, or bleeding
  Torn, stained, or bloody underwear

Neglect
  Dehydration or malnutrition
  Poor hygiene
  Inappropriate dress
  Unattended physical or medical needs
  Extensive bedsores

Adapted from Kleinschmidt, K.C. 1997. Elder abuse: A review. *Annals of Emergency Medicine* 30:463–472 (Mosby), with permission.

REPORTING OF ABUSE

The prehospital health care provider should bear in mind that mandatory reporting of elder abuse raises certain ethical concerns and may not be of clear benefit. Patients' refusal of intervention is a significant barrier to elder abuse prevention. Mandatory reporting may violate a competent elder person's right to privacy and autonomy. It may even cause elder persons to avoid medical care if they fear embarrassing investigations or ultimately institutionalization. Many mandatory reporting laws are modeled after similar laws for reporting child abuse and domestic violence, and may not address issues of autonomy or neglect. Elder abuse requires its own specific statutes to be most effective and beneficial for the abused elder person.

All states have enacted adult protective service laws or statutes that address elder abuse. There is considerable variability in the type and scope of these laws, including definitions of abuse, types and ages of persons covered by state law, mandatory and voluntary reporting by specific professionals and nonprofessionals, immunity from reporting, penalties for failing to report suspected abuse, report-receiving agencies, investigating agencies, and types of services specified under these laws. It is recommended that the prehospital health care provider be familiar with the law or laws addressing elder abuse in the state(s) in which he or she practices.

Currently, 33 states and the District of Columbia use a single law to cover both domestic and institutional elder abuse. Sixteen states have two separate laws to address domestic and institutional elder abuse, and one state has three laws to address this issue. In most of these states, elder abuse is covered under a general Adult Protective Service Law, but 11 states have laws that are elder abuse specific. All but 6 states (Colorado, Illinois, North Dakota, Pennsylvania, South Dakota, and Wisconsin) have mandatory reporting requirements, and specify professionals who are mandated to report elder abuse to a state agency or authority. Mandatory reporters most commonly cited in elder abuse laws are social workers, physicians, nurses, police officers, dentists, and dental hygienists, but many state laws include a provision for other mandatory reporters. Although none of the current Adult Protective Laws specifically name emergency medical services personnel as mandatory reporters, many states include any "licensed health care providers or professionals" as mandatory reporters of elder abuse. Prehospital health care providers would fall within this category.

Approximately half of all states have elder abuse laws that identify voluntary reporters. *Voluntary reporters* are usually defined as any person who has knowledge of domestic or institutional abuse of an elder person. Thus, whether or not a state has a mandatory reporting requirement, anyone who has cause to believe that elder abuse has occurred may report it to the appropriate authorities. All states have either a mandatory requirement or a provision for voluntary reporting, and many states have both. In addition, the elder abuse laws of all states include immunity for reporters of suspected abuse, so reporters need not fear any legal consequences if they report a suspected case of elder abuse in good faith. Finally, although most state laws either require EMS personnel to report suspected elder abuse or include a provision for voluntary reporting, it is important for every prehospital health care provider to be aware of the exact expectations of the state in which he or she practices. If a prehospital health care provider is unsure about elder abuse laws in his or her state, and elder abuse is suspected, it is appropriate to report the suspected abuse to a social worker, physician, nurse, or police officer. A listing of individual state toll-free telephone numbers for reporting suspected elder abuse is provided in Table 17.5.

Interventions

The aim of intervention for victims of elder abuse is to protect the victim from continuing harm and provide the basis for a more enjoyable life. Although ultimately the final and lasting interventions are made by other health professionals, the prehospital health care professional may be the first health care provider to recognize an abusive situation, and appropriate reporting may be life saving.

If abuse or neglect is suspected, the prehospital health care provider has two duties: 1) to ensure the patient's safety; and 2) to report the suspected abuse. If an elder patient is at risk for physical harm, the immediate priority for the prehospital health care provider is to remove the patient from the abusive or dangerous situation. Patient safety is assured through immediate transfer to an appropriate medical facility, usually a hospital emergency department, but it may also be to a supervised senior center or to a physician's office. Any patient who is being transported *back home* to a situation that appears unsafe should be returned to the facility where the transport commenced.

Table 17.5. Statewide Toll-Free Numbers for Reporting Suspected Domestic and Institutional Elder Abuse

Alabama	800-458-7214
Alaska	800-478-4444
Arizona	
Arkansas	800-482-8049
California	800-231-4024
Colorado	
Connecticut	800-443-9946
Delaware	800-223-9074
District of Columbia	202-727-2345
Florida	800-962-2873
Georgia	
Hawaii	
Idaho	
Illinois	800-252-8966
Indiana	800-992-6978
Iowa	800-362-2178
Kansas	800-922-5330
Kentucky	800-752-6200
Louisiana	800-259-4990
Maine	800-452-1990
Maryland	800-332-6347
Massachusetts	800-922-2275
Michigan	800-882-6066
Minnesota	
Mississippi	800-222-8880
Missouri	800-392-0210
Montana	406-332-6100
Nebraska	800-652-1999
Nevada	
New Hampshire	800-852-3345
New Jersey	800-624-4262
New Mexico	
New York	
North Carolina	
North Dakota	
Ohio	800-342-0553
Oklahoma	800-522-3511
Oregon	800-232-3020
Pennsylvania	
Rhode Island	800-322-2880
South Carolina	
South Dakota	
Tennessee	
Texas	800-254-5400
Utah	
Vermont	800-564-1612

Table 17.5. Continued

Virginia	
Washington	800-562-6078
West Virginia	800-352-6513
Wisconsin	
Wyoming	800-457-3659

The next priority for the prehospital health care provider who has encountered an abusive situation is to report the suspected elder abuse to the appropriate agency. The prehospital health care provider should make every effort to comply with reporting laws. The elder patient should also be informed that a report is being made on their behalf. It should be emphasized to the patient that reporting efforts are intended to increase their access to community services. Contact is made to the appropriate agency directly or through social services agencies. Agencies that investigate suspected cases of elder abuse and neglect include adult protective services, departments on aging, and law enforcement. Social services are usually available in hospital emergency departments or senior centers. If no social services are available at the time of transfer to the emergency department, a nurse or physician should be informed directly. Reporting to law enforcement agencies may also be required if the suspected abuse (physical or sexual) is considered a crime. Cases of suspected elder abuse occurring at a nursing home or other institutionalized setting should be reported to the appropriate state agency or to a social services agency independent of the institution involved. Any reporting of suspected abuse should be documented on the prehospital run-sheet.

Long-term intervention is beyond the scope of the practice of the prehospital health care provider, and usually involves the coordinated efforts of social workers, nurses, physicians, and administrators. A home visit is often necessary to assess the elder patient's living environment and ability to perform activities of daily living, such as walking, transferring, eating, bathing, and toileting. As these factors are often difficult to assess once the patient has arrived at the emergency department, it must be emphasized that the prehospital health care provider, even if in a patient's home for only a few minutes, can play a significant role in early identification of suspected elder abuse. Long-term intervention in cases of abuse does not always result in nursing home placement or disrupted family relationships. The most effective methods for combating elder abuse include in-home services, respite care, and improved coordination of community services. Assistance with functional independence is important in reducing an elder person's risk for abuse or neglect and can significantly improve quality of life.

Finally, long-term intervention in elder abuse involves education and training of prehospital health care providers, other health care professionals, fire and police officers, social services agencies, criminal justice professionals, and the public on the detection, assessment, and treatment of elder abuse. Public and professional awareness is the single most important factor in identifying cases of elder abuse.

In summary, elder abuse includes physical, emotional, financial, and sexual abuse as well as neglect and self-neglect. Millions of elder persons are abused every year, and this number is likely to increase as the population of elder persons increases. The prehospital health care provider can be instrumental in the identification of suspected elder abuse. If elder abuse is suspected, the prehospital health care provider should immediately remove the patient from harm, transport to a medical facility, and report the suspected abuse to the appropriate agency.

REVIEW QUESTIONS

1. All of the following are possible reasons that elder abuse may have increased over the past few decades *except*
   a. expansion of the elder population
   b. higher divorce rates
   c. increased prevalence of substance abuse in the younger population
   d. increase in the percentage of women working outside the home

2. Persons who are likely to commit elder abuse include all of the following *except*
   a. family members
   b. neighbors
   c. live-in caregivers
   d. nursing home staff

3. All of the following are risk factors for abuse in an elder person *except*
   a. mental illness
   b. frailty
   c. dementia
   d. having many caregivers

4. All of the following are risk factors that make a caretaker more likely to abuse an elder person *except*
   a. male sex
   b. substance abuse
   c. financial dependence of the caregiver on the elder person
   d. mental illness

5. Elders are often reluctant to report or admit to mistreatment by caregivers because of
   a. embarrassment
   b. fear of later retaliation

c. removal from their homes with loss of independence
d. all of the above

6. Prehospital providers are in a better position to identify elder abuse than most other caregivers for all of the following reasons *except*
   a. they are able to search the elder person's home for clues
   b. they have regular contact with elders
   c. they can examine firsthand an elder person's living environment
   d. they can witness the interaction between the elder person and the caregiver

7. Elders who are victims of self-neglect
   a. will take corrective action if an unsafe situation is identified for them
   b. have usually been neglected by other caregivers
   c. are at risk for psychological abuse
   d. are unable to take corrective action for unsafe situations

8. Adult protective service laws and elder abuse statutes
   a. follow federal guidelines and are similar from state to state
   b. all have provisions for mandatory reporting of elder abuse
   c. all address only persons over the age of 65
   d. vary from state to state

9. Mandatory reporters of elder abuse commonly cited in elder abuse statutes include all *except*
   a. social workers
   b. licensed health care professionals
   c. clergy
   d. police officers

10. If elder abuse or neglect is suspected, the prehospital provider is obligated to
    a. protect the patient from further harm
    b. move the patient to a safe location
    c. report the suspected abuse
    d. all of the above

SUGGESTED READING

American Academy of Family Physicians, Committee on Aging. 1990. *Geriabuse: Understanding the risks*. Kansas City: AAFP.

Gerson, L. W. and L. Schvarch. 1982. Emergency medical services utilization by the elderly. *Annals of Emergency Medicine* 11(11):610–612.

Gerson, L. W., D. T. Schelble, and J. E. Wilson. 1992. Using paramedics to identify at-risk elderly. *Annals of Emergency Medicine* 21(6):688–691.

18

Advance Directives in Medical Care

Robert Partridge, MD, MPH

OBJECTIVES

By the end of this chapter, the prehospital health care provider should be able to:

1 Define and recognize advance directives, living wills, do-not-resuscitate (DNR) orders, and durable powers of attorney.

2 Identify when to implement advance directives in medical care.

You are called to the home of an elder man with difficulty breathing. On arrival, you find the patient in severe respiratory distress. His respiratory rate is 40, heart rate is 140 and irregular, and blood pressure is 96/60. You note that he can speak only one word at a time, and his lips are cyanotic. He is using his accessory muscles to breathe, and chest wall retractions are present. As you administer oxygen, establish an IV, and place him on a cardiac monitor, he continues to deteriorate. As you prepare to intubate, the patient's daughter rushes in and identifies herself to you. She informs you that the patient "does not want to be put on a respirator." What should you do now? What are the ethical and legal concerns for the prehospital provider in this situation? How can you justify what you should (or should not) do?

ADVANCE DIRECTIVES

Advance directives in medical care are instructions given by patients to medical providers that define the extent of medical intervention desired in the event of acute illness or incapacitation. The basis for the development and acceptance of advance directives is that a patient has the right to self-determination concerning resuscitation or heroic intervention. Advance directives include living wills, durable powers of attorney, and DNR orders.

In 1990, the Patient Self Determination Act required that hospitals and nursing homes participating in the Medicare program record advance directives in medical care on all patients at the time of admission. Initially, advance directives were applicable only in the hospital setting, but as EMS personnel frequently make invasive life-saving interventions, advance directives are now playing a role in the prehospital arena. In the elder population, increasing numbers of people may have prepared advance directives that may directly affect the care administered by the prehospital health care provider.

The elder population is the group most likely to present the prehospital provider with an advance directive. This is because elders are more likely to have acute and chronic medical conditions and many have given some thought to what kinds of care they want if they are near death. In addition, to control health care costs, patients are cared for outside the hospital as often as possible. This means that more elders and chronically ill patients are cared for in nursing or residential facilities, or at home with assistance. Patients who are terminally ill and want no further intervention except to be kept comfortable during the dying process may be in hospice care. As a result, the likelihood of a prehospital critical illness or cardiac arrest is increased. Thus, it is imperative that prehospital providers be fully aware of the various types of advance directives that they may encounter so that unwanted care is not inadvertently provided.

Living Wills

All 50 states have legislation authorizing the use of advance directives. The Living Will is the most common type of advance directive recognized by states. Living Wills allow patients to specify under what conditions they would want care withheld or withdrawn. Typically, Living Wills cover a patient's desires in the event of terminal illness or permanent mental or physical incapacitation. Interventions such as whether the patient would want surgical procedures, medications, intravenous fluids, parenteral (IV) feedings, tube feedings, or other interventions that may prolong life but not necessarily improve the quality of life are described in Living Wills. For many patients, the specific interventions desired are often dependent on the likelihood of a good or bad outcome. Living Wills are not often considered in the prehospital setting because it is usually not possible to know if the directives are applicable or relevant. If a patient has a Living Will, it does not guarantee that a terminal condition exists, and might state that "in the event of" terminal illness, no life support should be instituted. Unless a specific DNR order is also stated, it may be impossible for the prehospital health care provider to quickly determine whether advanced life support measures should be instituted.

Durable Powers of Attorney

Durable Powers of Attorney are advance directives prepared by individuals that allow a surrogate (usually a family member or guardian) to exercise the advance directives outlined in a patient's Living Will. These are written documents that should be clearly stated, and if applicable, shown to the senior prehospital health care provider at the scene. Provided the prehospital health care provider can verify that the person presenting the documents is the person with power of attorney and acting in good faith, then the prehospital health care provider has a duty to fulfill the requests of the person with power of attorney on the patient's behalf. If a patient's wishes in an acute life-threatening situation are not known or not clear to the power of attorney, the prudent approach is for the prehospital health care provider to initiate appropriate advanced life support measures and seek guidance from medical control.

RETURNING TO THE CASE

This patient is incapacitated by his current acute medical condition and is unable to verbally communicate his wishes about aggressive resuscitation measures. You realize that unless aggressive measures are taken, he will soon be in cardiac arrest. The daughter is able to produce a valid written document, signed by the patient, stating what medical intervention he wants and under what conditions. The document states that he does not want to remain on a respirator if it is determined that he has an *irreversible* medical condition. However, it is clear that if a potentially reversible condition exists, then he wants all necessary measures taken. In conjunction with the medical control physician, you decide that his condition is probably reversible, and that it is likely that once the acute deterioration in respiratory status has been corrected, he will not need to remain on the ventilator. You are able to successfully intubate him at the scene, and his cardiovascular status stabilizes during transport.

DNR Orders

DNR orders are the most commonly known advance directives, and are frequently encountered in the elder population. DNR orders are orders of resuscitative management that apply to a patient when death is imminent, such as in severe shock, respiratory failure, or cardiac arrest. DNR orders usually indicate that a patient does not want any heroic measures to preserve life when death is imminent. These measures include intubation, defibrillation, cardiopulmonary resuscitation, and aggressive blood pressure management. Some or all of these measures may be selected by the patient. The specifics of the DNR order should be clearly stated and communicated to the prehospital health care provider. DNR orders are usually chosen by a patient who is known to be terminally or chronically ill.

The DNR order is the most common advance directive the prehospital health care provider is likely to encounter, especially in the elder population. There are two major problems associated with the implementation of the DNR order in the prehospital setting. The first is the problem of communicating the DNR order to the prehospital health care provider in a timely fashion, especially as the patient may be incapacitated and unable to do so. Documentation of DNR orders may also be inadequate or unavailable for the prehospital health care provider to review. Relatives or bystanders may be ignorant of a patient's wishes or may not be able to state the patient's exact wishes.

Methods used to identify a patient's DNR orders or advance directives vary according to regional and local protocols. Some states have successfully encouraged patients to wear colored wrist bands to communicate advance directives to prehospital providers. Other states, as well as some local providers, recognize documents that have been prepared in advance and are kept in a particular place in the home or have been previously communicated to the local ambulance service or fire department. These documents are instructions for the prehospital health care provider not to undertake certain specific interventions. To be effective, any such documents should be recognizable, consistent, clearly stated, and legally acceptable. These documents should also be familiar to the prehospital providers and specific with regard to the interventions to be given and those to be withheld. Methods such as these have had some success in practice, but are not currently in widespread use.

The second problem is the difficulty associated with implementing the DNR order in the prehospital setting. Although most prehospital providers are familiar with advance directives (usually DNR orders), many are uncomfortable implementing them and frequently defer that decision to hospital personnel. Prehospital providers have cited several reasons for their reluctance to implement advance directives. The greatest obstacle is fear of legal consequences. Other reasons include personal difficulty withholding care they are trained to provide, and ambiguity in the advance directives received. Specific statutes authorizing the implementation of advance directives in the prehospital setting have become more widespread in recent years. In 1992, only 11 states had such legislation in place. Currently, at least 25 states have either specific legislation authorizing implementation of advance directives in the prehospital setting or have attorney general opinions on record that prehospital advance directives are legally enforceable. Attorney general opinions do not have the force of law, but are used by courts as guidelines in interpreting existing law. The states with such legislation or attorney general opinions are listed in Table 18.1.

In many areas, local protocols exist to guide prehospital personnel on the implementation of advance directives in the field. Some private ambulance services also have specific policies on this issue. It is important for the prehospital health care provider to familiarize him- or herself with the laws and protocols applicable where he or she practices. Medical control, if available, may also be useful in interpreting advance directives or clarifying actions to be taken or withheld by the prehospital health care provider. If a significant doubt exists about the content, applicability, or authenticity of the advance directive, treat the patient according to standard prehospital protocols. Remember that just as the prehospital health care provider can be liable for *not* intervening to save a life, it is possible that he or she may be liable *for* intervening when such intervention

Table 18.1. States with Specific Legislation or Attorney General Opinions Authorizing Implementation of Advance Directives in the Prehospital Setting

Arkansas	North Carolina
Arizona	New Hampshire
California	New Jersey
Colorado	New Mexico
Connecticut	New York
Florida	Rhode Island
Georgia	South Carolina
Idaho	Tennessee
Illinois	Texas
Kansas	Virginia
Maryland	Washington
Montana	West Virginia

is not wanted. A strong understanding of these issues not only results in optimum patient care according to the patient's own wishes, but also in protection for the prehospital health care provider by adherence to the local or regional standard of care.

CASE OUTCOME

After arrival in the emergency department, the patient is diagnosed with a pulmonary embolism as the result of a venous clot in his right leg and is placed on IV heparin. He is admitted to the intensive care unit and is extubated after 3 days. The remainder of his hospital course is uneventful, and he is discharged home on warfarin (Coumadin®) on the seventh hospital day. After discharge, his daughter makes sure a copy of the patient's advance directives are on file with the local EMS provider, his doctor, and in an obvious place in his home.

SUMMARY

In summary, advance directives allow individuals to specify the extent of medical intervention desired at some future time. Advance directives include living wills, durable powers of attorney, and DNR orders. The DNR order is the advance directive most commonly encountered by the prehospital health care provider, usually in the elder population. Prehospital health care providers should familiarize themselves with state and local protocols covering the implementation of advance directives in the prehospital setting. If advance directives are implemented appropriately in the field, unwanted medical intervention can be avoided.

REVIEW QUESTIONS

1. All of the following are true about advance directives in medical care *except*
   a. They define the extent of medical care desired in the event of illness or incapacitation.
   b. They include living wills, durable powers of attorney, and DNR orders.
   c. Elders are the most likely to present advance directives to prehospital providers.
   d. They are valid only in the hospital.

2. Living Wills can be difficult to interpret or implement in the field because
   a. They may be too extensive and take too much time to read.
   b. They are not valid in every state.
   c. In the prehospital setting, it is difficult to know if the provisions of the Living Will are applicable or relevant to the prehospital phase of a patient's care.
   d. They usually cannot be found.
   e. All of the above.

3. All of the following are true about durable powers of attorney *except*
   a. They can be implemented in the field only if the patient is unresponsive.
   b. They allow another person to exercise the advance directives prepared by the patient.
   c. They should be accepted only by the prehospital provider if they are in writing and if the person presenting them has power of attorney.
   d. If the prehospital provider is in doubt about the terms or the validity of the durable power of attorney, then he or she should follow standard care and resuscitation protocols.

4. All of the following are true about DNR orders *except*
   a. They are advance directives that the prehospital provider is most likely to encounter in the elder population.
   b. They refer to a patient's wishes about CPR, intubation, defibrillation, and aggressive blood pressure support when death is imminent.
   c. DNR patients do not require care at the advanced life support level.
   d. They may be difficult to communicate to the prehospital provider.

5. Prehospital providers may have difficulty implementing an elder patient's DNR order for all of the following reasons *except*
   a. They may be uncomfortable withholding care they have been trained to provide.
   b. DNR orders are not legal in most states.
   c. They may fear legal consequences.
   d. The DNR orders may not be stated clearly.

6. If in doubt about how to implement a patient's DNR order, the prehospital care provider should
   a. disregard the orders and provide the applicable standard of care
   b. implement the order as he or she sees fit
   c. transfer the patient to the nearest medical facility without any intervention
   d. consult the medical control physician

SUGGESTED READING

Adams, J. and A. B. Wolfson. 1990. Ethical issues in geriatric emergency medicine. *Emergency Medicine Clinics of North America* 8(2):183–191.

Adams, J. 1993. Prehospital do-not-resuscitate orders: A survey of state policies in the United States. *Prehospital and Disaster Medicine* 8(4):317–322.

Partridge, R. A., A. Virk, A. Sayah, and R. Antosia. 1998. Field experience with prehospital advance directives. *Annals of Emergency Medicine* 32:589–593.

Index

Chest discomfort, 28–31
Chest, flail. *See* Flail chest
Chest pain, 25–28
    aortic dissection and, 26–27
    myocardial infarction as, 25
    pulmonary embolism, cause of, 27
Chest trauma, 13, 163–178
    aorta/great vessels, disruption of, with, 170–171
    assessment of, 171–174
    blunt trauma, type of, 163
    cardiac contusion as, 170
    cardiac tamponade as, 167–168
    causes of, 172
    chest wall and, 13
    clavicular fractures as, 169
    crepitation in, 173
    DCAP-BTLS for, 173
    flail chest, type of, 163–164
    hemothorax as, 167
    immediate intervention for, 163
    kyphosis in, 166
    monitoring and stabilization of, 165–166
    pneumothorax as, 166–167
    pulmonary contusion as, 169
    rib fractures as, 168–169
    stabilization/treatment of, 175–178
    statistics on, 163
    sternal fractures as, 169
    tension pneumothorax as, 167
    tracheobronchial injuries as, 170
    traumatic asphyxia as, 1668
Chest wounds, open
    treatment of, 176–177
CHF (congestive heart failure), 9, 30, 31, 207, 215, 216
    COPD, appears identical to, 31
    coronary artery disease as cause of, 31
    Dobutamine for, 33
    Dopamine for, 33
    dyspnea and, 31
    hypertension as cause of, 31
    hypotension, symptom of, 30
    medications for, 33
    morphine for, 33
    Nitroglycerine for, 33
    Nitroprusside for, 33
    Norepinephrine for, 33
    rales with, 31
Cholangitis, ascending, 61
Chronic obstructive pulmonary disease. *See* COPD
Circulation, 10–11
    pulses and, 10–11
Clavicular fracture, 169
CNS (central nervous system), 34, 78
    atrophy, brain mass and, 78
    decreased nerve conduction time of, 78
    dysfunction of, 34–35
    heat exhaustion and functioning of, 126

    syncope and, 34–35
    TIA and, 78
CO (carbon monoxide), 91, 131
CO_2 (carbon dioxide), 43, 46
Cognitive difficulties, 7, 8, 9
    CNS and, 78
    delirium and, 138
    depression and, 140
Colle's fracture, 196
Coma. *See* Unresponsiveness
Confusion, 89
Congestive heart failure. *See* CHF
Consciousness, disorders of, 86
Constipation, 55, 60
COPD (chronic obstructive pulmonary disease), 31, 43–46, 131, 144, 193
    albuterol for, 46
    asthma in, 44–45
    CHF appears identical to, 31
    chronic bronchitis in, 44
    emphysema in, 43–44
    ipratroprium bromide for, 46
    oxygen for, 46
    pneumothorax and, 50
    symptoms of, 45
    treatment modalities for, 46
    tripod stance with, 45
Crepitation, chest trauma and,173
CVA (cerebrovascular accident), 79
    stroke, same as, 79

DCAP-BTLS (Deformities, Contusions, Abrasions, Penetrations/Punctures, Burns, Tenderness, Lacerations, Swelling), 173. *See also* Chest trauma
Deep venous thrombosis. *See* DVT
Delirium, 89, 136, 137–138
    assessment of, 142–144
    causes of, 90, 138
    dementia, compared with, 138–139
    missing the diagnosis of, 138
    overmedication (polypharmacy), cause of, 137
    risk factors for, 138
    symptoms of, 90, 142–143
    underdiagnosis of, 137
Delirium tremens. *See* DTs
Dementia, 89, 136, 230
    assessment of, 142–144
    delirium, compared with, 138
    irreversible causes of, 136
    reversible causes of, 136
    symptoms of, 142–143
Dentures, 9–10
Depression, 139–140
    medical causes of, 140
    reactive, 139
    suicide and, 139
    symptoms of, 139–140

TIA (transient ischemic attack) (*continued*)
  seizures and, 83
  stroke with, 79, 80, 81
Toxicologic exposure
  activated charcoal for, 113
  adverse drug/toxin reactions and, 111–112
  assessment of, 113–114
  drug implications in, 111
  etiologies of, 110–111
  gastric lavage for, 113–114
  ipecac for, 113
  materials, hazardous and, 113
  poison ingestion and 113
  SAMPLE history in, 114
  social/environmental factors and, 111
  treatment for, 115–117
Tracheobronchial injuries, 170
  paper bag syndrome and, 170
  treatment of, 177
Transient ischemic attack. *See* TIA
Transporting/stabilizing elder patients, 17–18
Trauma. *See* Abdominal/pelvic trauma; Blunt
      trauma; Chest trauma; Head/neck trauma;
      Musculoskeletal trauma
Traumatic asphyxia, 168, 176
Tripod stance, 45
Tunica adventitia, 26
Tunica intima, 26
Tunica media, 26

Ulcer, peptic, 57–58
  NSAIDs and, 57
Unresponsiveness (coma), 86–89
  AEIOU–TIPS, used in evaluation of, 87
  airway in, 88
  AVPU, useful for describing, 86, 88
  bradycardia and, 89
  cervical spine in, 88
  consciousness, levels of with, 86
  diabetic, 99
  DKA, 100
  eyes, examine with, 89
  hyperosmolar hyperglycemic, 101–102
  hypertension and, 89

hypoglycemic, 102–103
myxadema, 105
naloxone for, 88
narcotic overdose and, 88
skin examination during, 89
Urinary retention, 71–72
  atypical, 72
  BPH in, 71
  medications and, 71–72
Urinary tract infection. *See* UTI
Uterine prolapse, 70
UTI (urinary tract infection), 67–68
  DM and, 68
  epididymitis/orchitis as, 69
  phimosis/paraphimosis in, 70
  priapism as, 70
  prostate disease and, 67–68, 69
  treatment, possible for, 68

Vaginal bleeding, 73
  sexual assault and, 73
Valente, Jonathan H., 108
Valsalva maneuver, 85
Vancomycin-resistant *Enterococcus*. *See* VRE
Vasodepressor syncope, 35
Vasovagal syncope, 35, 85
VBI (vertebrobasilar insufficiency), 34–35
Ventilation
  assisted, 13
  bag–valve mask, 10
Ventolin, 47
Verapamil, 208–209
Vertebral fracture, 194-195
Vertebrobasilar insufficiency. *See* VBI
Vital signs, 15–16, 31
  changes in, 24
  four basic, 15
Voluntary reporters, 235
VRE (vancomycin-resistant *Enterococcus*), 49

Wernicke's syndrome, 138, 141
Williams, Mark, 42
Wilson, Brian, 134
Wolf–Parkinson–White syndrome, 211